THE SAVVY
MEDICAL
CONSUMER

OTHER BOOKS FROM
THE PEOPLE'S MEDICAL SOCIETY

Getting the Most for Your Medical Dollar

Massage Made Easy

Medicare Made Easy

Medicine on Trial

Misdiagnosis: Woman As a Disease

So You're Going to Be a Mother

Take This Book to the Gynecologist With You

Take This Book to the Hospital With You

Take This Book to the Pediatrician With You

The Complete Book of Relaxation Techniques

Yoga Made Easy

Your Medical Rights

THE SAVVY MEDICAL CONSUMER

By Charles B. Inlander
and
The Staff of the People's Medical Society

≣People's Medical Society®

Allentown, Pennsylvania

The People's Medical Society is a nonprofit consumer health organization dedicated to the principles of better, more responsive and less expensive medical care. Organized in 1983, the People's Medical Society puts previously unavailable medical information into the hands of consumers so that they can make informed decisions about their own health care.

Membership in the People's Medical Society is $20 a year and includes a subscription to the *People's Medical Society Newsletter.* For information, write to the People's Medical Society, 462 Walnut Street, Allentown, PA 18102, or call 610-770-1670.

This and other People's Medical Society publications are available for quantity purchase at discount. Contact the People's Medical Society for details.

© 1997 by the People's Medical Society
Printed in the United States of America

Library of Congress Cataloging-in-Publication Data

Inlander, Charles B.
      The savvy medical consumer / by Charles B. Inlander
and the staff of the People's Medical Society.
         p. cm.
     ISBN 1-882606-31-0 (pbk.)
     1. Medical care. 2. Medical care—Cost control.
3. Consumer education. I. People's Medical Society (U.S.)
II. Title.
RA410.5.I55   1997
362.1—dc21   97-8923
                                               CIP

1 2 3 4 5 6 7 8 9 0
First printing, September 1997

CONTENTS

INTRODUCTION

It takes a savvy consumer to cut through the maze known as the American health-care system. But with the right information, the right attitude and a willingness to be just a little assertive, you can get quality health care at a cost far less than what many of your friends and neighbors pay.

Despite all its virtues, all its miracles and all its victories, our health-care system is fraught with physical and economic dangers. It is a system that even renowned medical experts have labeled "out of control."

There are 42 million Americans without health insurance. Another 30 million people are underinsured—they could not cover their medical bills if confronted with a major illness or a prolonged medical encounter. Corporations that once provided liberal health-care benefits to employees at little or no cost now require employees to pay part of their insurance premiums, deductibles and copayments. Some companies have even cut their benefits. Most have switched to managed-care programs, like health maintenance organizations (HMOs).

The numbers tell the story. In 1996, the United States spent 14.5 percent of its gross national product on health care. That's $1 trillion, or more than three times what we spent on national defense. It also represented a 5 percent increase over the previous year. Overall inflation for the same period was around 3 percent. And while health-care inflation has leveled off for the last several years, analysts predict it will start climbing again as baby boomers reach their 50s and start needing more medical services.

If those numbers don't hit home, try these. The average American household of four spends $14,000 each year for health-care services. This includes out-of-pocket payments to doctors and hospitals, insurance premiums, medical equipment purchases, federal and state taxes used for health care and the cost of health-care benefits built into the goods and services you buy.

Under normal economic circumstances, health-care costs should be going down. Demand is nowhere near the level of supply. Approximately 55 percent of the hospital beds in this country are empty. Every one of America's major cities has a doctor glut—many more doctors than we need in order to provide quality care to consumers. A coronary bypass, a procedure that has increased in frequency by more than 100 percent in the last 10 years, went from an average of $20,000 per procedure in 1980 to close to $50,000 in 1995. Yet in the 1970s, when that particular operation was coming into vogue, medical gurus were promising a dramatic drop in cost as the operation became more commonplace. That's a pretty serious medical misdiagnosis.

Even the quality of American medicine is coming into question. Hospital infections are rampant. One out of 10 people who enter a hospital today can expect to acquire an infection they did not have when they were admitted. That is an almost 100 percent increase in the last decade. Twenty percent of all people who enter a hospital acquire a condition while in the hospital that they did not have before they came. Several studies have shown that up to 40 percent of the people admitted to hospitals are there as a result of something a doctor has done to them.

Americans get the most health care in the world and pay the highest fees for it, yet overall the nation ranks relatively low, compared with other developed countries, in such categories as length of life and infant mortality.

As a result, consumers now are taking a more "buyer beware" attitude about medical services. We are questioning more, saying no to what appear to be useless or unnecessary services, seeking second opinions, using outpatient services and entering wellness and rehabilitation programs.

The federal government, insurers and businesses have implemented programs such as HMOs and other managed-care models that require patients to get preapproval for treatments to ensure that the consumer is getting the right treatment for the condition presented. Medicare beneficiaries are staying fewer days in the hospital than before and are being urged to join cost-saving Medicare HMOs. Insurance companies are encouraging the use of less costly outpatient services. Businesses are telling their employees to use fewer medical services and to use them only when absolutely necessary.

Yet medical inflation continues to outpace general inflation. And even with managed care becoming the predominant form of medical insurance, the number of uninsured continues to rise, the cost of care continues to go up, and the quality of care continues to be questionable. Hospitals are merging with one another to survive, with many moving from nonprofit to for-profit status. Insurers that were once nonprofit are also switching over to for-profit status. They all say it's to compete in this highly competitive market. But the bottom line for you is more cost and uncertain quality. And the bottom line for the hospitals and insurers is bigger profits than ever before.

The change in the health-care system has not only affected consumers, but it's also affected practitioners. Now they must answer to the payer, either a managed-care company, insurer, government or large employer. Until just a few years ago, doctors ruled the roost. They told payers how much a service would cost, and payers forked over the cash. Today payers negotiate fees and payments based on the volume of business they can send a doctor's way. And, despite all their yelling and screaming, doctors and other practitioners are cutting deals, while they still try to deny they are business types.

They talk about caring, healing, touching and compassion. They tell us how hard and how long they work, about the sacrifices they make, and about the terrible trials and tribulations they endure in the service of the sick and needy. But consumers have come to understand that beneath the white coat, behind the surgical mask, between the two tubes of the stethoscope resides a businessperson. Consumers are asking for the information and tools to deal with these professionals in a businesslike way. In other words, consumers want medical accountability.

That is precisely why we wrote this book. Medicine is a business. While it is a business that deals with illness and the human condition, we must remember that economics is always at play. Every time we use medical services, there is a cost attached. Unless we have insurance, we may not be "accepted" by a hospital or doctor. Doctors have signs in their offices asking people to pay at the time of visit. Hospitals post notices about minimum fees for use of the emergency room. No matter how helpful a medical service may be, the business element is always involved.

For the past several years, there has been a movement among business and government to contain the cost of medical care. The reality is that the cost-containment strategies employed by business and government have been successful in containing costs—but only for some businesses and the federal government. They have had very little effect on the average consumer, employee or Medicare beneficiary. In fact, cost containment has not meant a reduction in fees, but rather a reduction in the amount of money spent by parties trying to contain their costs.

Thirty-two years ago, when the Medicare program was launched, Americans over the age of 65 were spending 15 percent of their incomes for medical services. That predicament was the impetus for passage of the Medicare legislation. Citizens were outraged at these costs, and the Medicare program came into being. By 1996, however, something astounding had occurred. Medicare beneficiaries were now spending upwards of 25 percent of their incomes on medical care over and above what Medicare covered. In other words, the very economic conditions that older people confronted in 1965 and that brought about Medicare were even worse in 1996.

So much for the bad news. Now, what do we do as medical consumers? First, we arm ourselves with information—facts and figures that help us find the best care at the best price. Second, we formulate the questions that will get us the substantive answers we need from our health-care providers.

Here's the good news. In the pages that follow, we have listed and explained hundreds of ways to be a savvy medical consumer. We have given you the facts and information that will help you find the best health care at the lowest price. Some of what you read, you may already know. Other ideas may never have dawned on you.

Every one of these tips to find quality health care and lower your health-care costs works. They have worked for others just like you.

As president of the People's Medical Society, I am convinced that as individuals we can have quality health care and keep our personal expenditures down. As I travel around the country speaking to tens of thousands of people each year, they tell me what they have done to reduce costs for themselves. We have listed those methods in this book.

This book is your key for entering the world of quality health care and reasonable medical costs. We have tried to give you real actions you can take to make sure you receive the best medical care at the best price. (And believe me, I know they work. I have tried many myself.)

The staff of the People's Medical Society and I have reviewed all of these ideas. They are winners. And you too can be a winner over medical incompetence and medical inflation.

Read these ideas carefully. Use them at the next appropriate time. You will be surprised at just how easy it is to take charge of your own medical care. Do not be intimidated by medical professionals when you confront them. Remember that they are in business and so are you. It is your business to get the best care at the lowest cost.

This book will help you do that.

Charles B. Inlander
President
People's Medical Society

Terms printed in boldface can be found in the glossary, beginning on page 121. Only the first mention of the word in the text will be boldfaced.

We have tried to use male and female pronouns in an egalitarian manner throughout this book. Any imbalance in usage has been in the interest of readability.

Doctors

Doctors are the so-called gatekeepers of the medical world. Through them, you enter the worlds of the hospital, laboratory and pharmacy. But doctors are also much more. Not only do they determine the quantity of health care you receive and often set the price, but they're also responsible for the quality of care you receive. Even with the advent of **managed care**, doctors control most aspects of the health-care delivery system, including what services you'll receive and where you'll receive them. For these reasons—and more personal ones as well—you'll want to develop a good working relationship with your doctor. Knowing how to interact with a doctor makes you a smarter consumer, improving your prospects of getting high-quality care. By working carefully and assertively with your practitioner, you can increase your chances of receiving high-quality medical care and greatly lower your health costs.

First things first—how do you go about looking for Dr. Right? The fact of the matter is that most consumers spend more time selecting a roofer than they do choosing someone to look after their health. Choosing a doctor isn't easy. It's a process filled with questions, both for the pros-

13

pective doctor and for yourself, but the savvy consumer will realize that the right choice will save money and perhaps even a life.

Begin your search by getting a few good recommendations from family members, friends and neighbors. Word of mouth is still one of the best methods of finding out which doctors are taking new patients and what others think of those doctors. The old adage "If you want to find a good doctor, ask a nurse" is probably a good one but not always practical. And don't overlook your present doctor, especially if your relationship with this doctor is ending because he is leaving practice or retiring. Ask him for names of other practitioners to consider. Here are some other sources that may help you find a doctor:

▶ *Doctor referral services operated by a local medical society (usually county-based).* Not necessarily our first choice, such services will refer only those doctors who are members of the society.

▶ *Hospital-sponsored physician referral services.* Similar to medical society referral services, in this case a local hospital refers you to a list of physicians who are either on its staff or have privileges at its facility. Neither referral service will comment on the specific ability of referred physicians other than to perhaps mention any **board certifications**.

▶ *Newspaper advertisements of doctors announcing the opening of a new practice.* Be wary, however, and ask yourself why the doctor is advertising. Is it to attract patients because she is just out of medical school? Or is in a highly competitive and glutted market? Or has just moved in from a state where her license was revoked?

▶ *Your company personnel office.* Ask if your company maintains a list of doctors other employees have recommended.

▶ *Your health insurance company.* Check if your insurer has any local doctors to recommend or if it recommends **specialists** for particular conditions.

▶ *Listings in the telephone directory.* Doctors' names are usually arranged according to practice or specialty, but be aware that just because a doctor says she specializes in a certain area of medicine does not mean the doctor actually took any advanced training in it. A doctor can practice in any specialty area she chooses.

▶ *Senior centers.* Some have referral services.

▶ *Your managed-care company.* If you are enrolled in a managed-care program, such as a **health maintenance organization (HMO)**, it will have a list of doctors from which you must choose (see also chapter 6).

Here now are some savvy tips for dealing with doctors.

◆ *Check for board certification.*

Physicians who are board certified have to meet additional training requirements and must pass a rigorous examination administered by a specialty board. Since a large difference in fees between certified and noncertified physicians is unlikely, you may as well go with the doctor who has additional training—*if* he indeed does. Physicians know that consumers have become more savvy about credentials, so they're doing everything they can to make themselves look better. So be alert to physicians who play a little game by putting initials after their names. They're counting on your being impressed when you see the initials "B.E." following their names. Don't be; it only means "board eligible."

Another favorite ploy of some physicians is to list themselves as board certified but fail to tell you in which specialty. You have to make sure that the physician is board certified in his main field of practice. To check the board-certification status of a physician, call the American Board of Medical Specialties. The group's toll-free number is 800-776-CERT. (When you call, have at hand the physician's full name and his city and state.)

◆ *Ask for a get-acquainted visit.*

Before you seek the professional services of a new doctor, we suggest that you contact several physicians to determine if they are accepting new patients. If they are, set up a short get-acquainted visit and offer to pay for the time. (We've seen surveys of physicians showing a range between $30 and $60 for such get-acquainted visits. If a particular doctor wants more, negotiate [tell him the range we quote]. Some physicians may not charge you for the time, but always offer to pay; it's one investment that will return dividends.) The purpose of this visit is to find out if you and the doctor see eye to eye on health issues and if her office services are efficient, and to have any of your questions answered *before* you commit to her services. No matter how thorough your doctor-shopping expedition has been, many problems do not arise until the first face-to-face encounter with the practitioner and the office staff, but with a get-acquainted visit, your chances of things going wrong are lowered.

◆ *Check fees in advance.*

There is a surprising amount of variation in basic fees, and indeed, doctors tend not to publish or post their fees for a variety of reasons. The primary one is that they do not have a set fee for a given procedure. (The skeptic would say that the fees doctors charge have nothing to do with their qualifications—they are more likely to be due to the size of the doctor's mortgage or car payment.)

Each time you visit the doctor, ask what the charges will be for the procedures, tests and treatments the doctor will perform. If the doctor does not know what his fees are, then insist that the person who does know come into the room with you and the doctor. If you are in a managed-care program, such as an HMO, make sure you know if there is a **copayment** required each time you visit the doctor. This is common practice, with copayments ranging from $10 to $20 per visit.

◆ *Negotiate charges and fees.*

Most people never think of negotiating with a doctor. Negotiating is something we do with a car dealer or a flea-market vendor. The savvy consumer, however, never forgets that medicine is a business—in fact, the biggest business in America—and, therefore, normal business practices apply, including negotiation.

Generally, doctors are willing to lower their standard fees for patients with limited incomes or special economic circumstances. Mind you, doctors probably won't readily admit that they negotiate their fees, but in reality, they do. Every time a physician signs an insurance agreement, she is permitting someone else to set the price of service. Businesses have also taken actions that force employees to shop for the best price among physicians. By setting maximum reimbursement levels on insurance plans, businesses are telling employees to find the best value. Physicians are well aware of this practice and, because of increased competition, are more willing to adjust their fees in order to get the business.

Here's the strategy: If the quoted fee seems excessively high or is more than you can pay, tell the doctor. Indicate that you feel this is wrong or that you cannot afford such a cost. Ask if the fee can be lowered in your case or if some other payment scheme can be devised. If you have been using the physician for many years, call upon your loyal patronage. Remember that doctors' services are like airline fares: No two people are necessarily paying the same amount for the same class of service to the same destination. And just like the airlines, a doctor's financial security over the long haul is based on your repeat business.

◆ *Negotiate fees associated with a single problem.*

Have you ever been bugged by the doctor who charges you $50 to treat an ear infection and then charges another

$30 when you come back again two weeks later to check its status? You should be. Negotiate a single fee for the whole problem. Tell your doctor at the first visit that you believe the original fee should cover his second look. Obviously, if there is still a problem, you'll pay for it. But if the problem is gone, and the visit is just a minute or two, ask him to agree to no additional charge. Use this strategy as often as you can. For example, if you receive biweekly allergy shots, negotiate a fee that includes only the shot, not an office visit charge. If you need to have your blood pressure checked weekly, negotiate a low fee, maybe $5 instead of a regular office visit charge.

Even if you're insured, negotiate. The more money you save your insurance company, the less likely it is that your premiums will increase in the future.

◆ *Make it clear to your doctor that all tests must be specifically approved by you before ordering.*

Millions of medical tests are performed annually, and American consumers and insurers spend billions of dollars for them. Yet many millions of these tests aren't necessary, say some experts. And many of the tests aren't very accurate. Others have serious risks and iffy benefits. So you may well wonder, Should I have that test? Does my malady really require two or three tests to determine a **diagnosis**?

The savvy consumer *can* take charge and *can* minimize the risks and costs of unnecessary testing. Here's how:

▶ Ask why you need the test. Before you agree to any test, ask your doctor what will be done if the test results are abnormal *and* what will be done if the test results are normal.

▶ Ask how reliable the test is, what the chance is of a false-positive or false-negative result and how risks of either can be minimized. (A false-positive result means that the test shows up positive, or abnormal, but no disease is actually present. A false-negative result means that the test shows up negative, or normal, but you actually have the disease.) Mind you, no test is 100 percent accurate, but you should be told the usefulness and the limits of tests if you are to make an informed decision.

▶ Find out what alternatives you have if you refuse the test.

▶ Ask how much the test will cost. And don't forget to check with your insurance company prior to undergoing an expensive test to see if it will cover the total cost.

◆ *Discuss all options before agreeing to tests.*

Doctors have come to rely on tests to such an extent that they tend to order them routinely, whether or not they're necessary to confirm a diagnosis. Discuss the necessity of each and every recommended test in detail with your doctor. Unnecessary medical testing, done solely as a defensive measure, costs consumers billions of dollars each year. Two Stanford University professors recently estimated the cost of **defensive medicine** at $50 billion per year!

Even in the area of testing, negotiation can play an important role. Let's assume the doctor recommends a particular test. Here's how to negotiate whether it is the most appropriate one for your current situation: Begin by asking, "Why this particular test?" Ask if there is a more comprehensive test that will answer more questions. Ask the doctor to explain the risks associated as well as matters like pain or time involved with the procedure. Of course, ask the price and be prepared to pinpoint whether that price is all-inclusive.

When you get all the information, sit down with the doctor and negotiate what you want. Don't be afraid to ask more questions or make decisions that are not necessarily what the doctor might have originally recommended. Make sure this is a give-and-take situation. Ask the doctor, "If I do X, what are my chances that Y will occur?" In other words, come to an agreement.

◆ *Check if the doctor uses an in-office laboratory.*

In-office labs tend to be less expensive, but just as with any commercial laboratory, the test results are only as good as the people and equipment carrying out the test. Furthermore, regulations and standards governing in-office laboratories vary from state to state, and critics of office-based testing point to problems with accuracy, quality and quality control, lack of adequately trained laboratory staff and staff turnover— and incentive to profit through overtesting. Study after study shows small in-office laboratories tend to have a greater variability in test results than do large, regulated labs. Any one of these problems can take a toll on your health and finances.

So be sure to ask your doctor if her lab is inspected and certified. Find out the qualifications of the people working in the lab. What are their credentials? Is anyone a medical technologist, trained in the proper collection and preparation of specimens and the operation of the equipment? How often is the equipment inspected and calibrated, and when was the last time this was done? Here are four organizations that certify laboratories:

American Society of Clinical Pathologists
2100 W. Harrison St.
Chicago, IL 60612

College of American Pathologists
325 Waukegan Rd.
Northfield, IL 60093

Commission on Office Laboratory Accreditation
8701 Georgia Ave., Suite 610
Silver Spring, MD 20910

National Accrediting Agency for Clinical
      Laboratory Sciences
8410 W. Bryn Mawr Ave., Suite 670
Chicago, IL 60631

In 1983, the People's Medical Society created the Code of Practice as a statement we believe each doctor should subscribe to. Ask your doctor to review it and tell you whether he will apply it to your care.

THE PEOPLE'S MEDICAL SOCIETY CODE OF PRACTICE

I will assist you in finding information resources, support groups and health-care providers to help you maintain and improve your health. When you seek my care for specific problems, I will abide by the following Code of Practice:

I. Office Procedures

1. I will post or provide a printed schedule of my fees for office visits, procedures, tests and surgery and provide **itemized bills**.

2. I will provide certain hours each week when I will be available for nonemergency telephone **consultation**.

3. I will schedule appointments to allow the necessary time to see you with minimal waiting. I will promptly report test results to you and return phone calls.

4. I will allow and encourage you to bring a friend or relative into the examining room with you.

5. I will facilitate your getting your medical and hospital records and will provide you with copies of your test results.

II. Choice in Diagnosis and Treatment

1. I will let you know your prognosis, including whether your condition is terminal or will cause disability or pain, and will explain why I believe further diagnostic activity or treatment is necessary.

continued on next page

THE PEOPLE'S MEDICAL SOCIETY
CODE OF PRACTICE
continued

2. I will discuss with you diagnostic, treatment and medication options for your particular problem (including the option of no treatment) and describe in understandable terms the risk of each alternative, the chances of success, the possibility of pain, the effect on your functioning, the number of visits each would entail and the cost of each alternative.

3. I will describe my qualifications to perform the proposed diagnostic measures or treatments.

4. I will let you know of organizations, support groups and medical and lay publications that can assist you in understanding, monitoring and treating your problem.

5. I will not proceed until you are satisfied that you understand the benefits and risks of each alternative and I have your agreement on a particular course of action.

◆ *Make it clear to your doctor that all consultations with other physicians must be specifically approved by you before ordering.*

Especially during periods of hospitalization, you may find yourself being billed by specialists for consultations that you may not even have known took place, much less that you approved. Also, check with your insurance company or employee benefits office before agreeing to any consultations; some companies require precertification, which means that the service, the consultation or even the test must be approved in advance. Failure to get prior approval could reduce your benefit and result in a large out-of-pocket expense for you.

◆ Buy a medical guide to aid you in deciding whether to see a doctor.

There are several good home medical guides available that offer clear advice and instructions for determining whether a doctor's care is necessary. These are just a few such guides:

The American Medical Association Family Medical Guide 3rd rev. ed. Edited by Jeffrey R. M. Kuntz, M.D., and Asher J. Finkel, M.D. (New York: Random House, 1994).

Doctor in the House: Your Best Guide to Effective Medical Self-Care. John C. Herbert, M.D. (Totowa, NJ: Humana Press, 1994).

Mayo Clinic Family Health Book rev. ed. Edited by David E. Larson, M.D. (New York: William Morrow, 1996).

Self-Care: Your Family Guide to Symptoms and How to Treat Them. Don R. Powell, Ph.D. (Allentown, PA: People's Medical Society, 1996).

Take Care of Yourself: Your Personal Guide to Self-Care and Preventing Illness 5th ed. Donald M. Vickery, M.D., and James F. Fries, M.D. (Reading, MA: Addison-Wesley, 1993).

◆ Do not use a specialist as a primary-care physician.

A primary-care physician is one who cares for the whole patient and has not specialized in any one area of the body or condition. Adults have three types of primary-care physicians from which to choose:

▶ **General practitioners.** Though dwindling in numbers, there are still some general practitioners in practice today.

▶ **Family practitioners.** Doctors who intend to become F.P.'s take additional training beyond medical school—a three-year residency that covers certain aspects of internal medicine, gynecology, minor surgery, obstetrics, pediatrics, orthopedics and preventive medicine—and then must pass a comprehensive examination.

▶ *Internists.* Like family practitioners, these doctors complete a three-year residency and must pass a comprehensive examination, but they do not normally take training in pediatrics, orthopedics and obstetrics. Instead, they have more advanced training in diagnosis and management of problems involving areas such as the gastrointestinal system, the heart, the kidney, the liver and the endocrine system.

If you require the care of a specialist for a specific problem (such as a cardiologist for a heart problem), do not ask that person to treat any problems not related to that particular specialty. Not only are a specialist's time and care more expensive, but he may not be the best qualified to deal with problems outside of his specific area of expertise.

◆ *Always go to a nonspecialist first— specialists are rarely necessary.*

As you can see from the previous item, primary-care physicians are able to treat the vast majority of illnesses, and they will readily refer you to a specialist if necessary. But in the meantime, you will have paid less for the care you received. Furthermore, self-referral to a specialist has potential problems. Sure, at some time or another, any of us may need a specialist to help discover the cause of a troublesome problem or to manage an uncommon or complicated disease; however, out of the obvious need for experts in fields of medicine has come an overspecialized, fragmented system of medical care. And out of this has sprung the phenomenon of, for example, the orthopedist who sees "the back problem" and not the person as a whole, the urologist who sees "the bladder infection" and not the person's complete medical condition and so on. Specialization profoundly influences the way medicine is practiced. Too often, patients are referred from doctor to doctor to be reassured that nothing is wrong with the organ system of the doctor's field of interest or specialty.

Self-refer only if you must and if you feel that you, alone or preferably with an **advocate** (a friend or relative) by your side, can maintain control over any decisions regarding tests, procedures and so on. But first determine what type of specialist you need, or even if you need one. Furthermore, if you belong to an HMO or **preferred-provider organization (PPO)** and decide to see a specialist *first*—in short, self-refer, a practice that HMOs and PPOs frown upon—you could be responsible for the entire cost of the visit.

WHAT IS A SPECIALIST?

A specialist is a doctor who concentrates on a specific body system, age group or disorder. After obtaining an M.D. (Doctor of Medicine) or D.O. (Doctor of Osteopathy) degree, a doctor then undergoes two to three years of supervised specialty training (called a **residency**). Many specialists also take one or more years of additional training (called a **fellowship**) in a specific area of their specialty (called a **subspecialty**).

How can you tell if a doctor is a trained specialist? A doctor who has taken extra training in his field often chooses to become board certified. In addition to the extra training, the doctor must pass a rigorous examination administered by a specialty board, a national board of professionals in that specialty field. A doctor who passes the board examination is given the status of *Diplomate*. Plus, most board-certified doctors become members of their medical specialty societies, and any doctor who meets the full requirements for membership is called a *Fellow* of the society and may use the designation. For instance, the title "FACOG" after a doctor's name denotes that she is a Fellow of the American College of Obstetricians and Gynecologists.

◆ *Demand itemized bills.*

Itemized bills are always a good idea because they let you know exactly what you are paying for and help you determine whether you are being billed for a service you did not receive. Sometimes, even an itemized bill doesn't give you enough information to make such determinations. Hospitals and doctors use esoteric codes; if such codes appear on your statement, without explanation, contact the business office and ask for a statement in plain English. If you are still not clear about a charge or have a dispute, ask your doctor to verify that a particular service, test or product was ordered for your care.

◆ *Use ambulatory-care centers (or walk-in/walk-out centers) rather than hospital emergency rooms if your doctor is not available.*

Anytime you feel you need a doctor's care, you should call your doctor first. But if your doctor is not available, an ambulatory-care center (sometimes called urgicenter or emergi-center) is usually less expensive and less time-consuming than a hospital emergency room (ER). Such facilities—either independent clinics or affiliated with hospitals—offer basic medical care on a walk-in basis for 12 or even 24 hours of the day, rather than only during traditional office hours. The mission in most primary/emergency/urgent-care centers is to treat minor injuries or short-term illnesses and provide immediate treatment for routine problems—for example, cuts, sprains, dislocated bones, sore throats and earaches.

◆ *Get a second opinion.*

First isn't always best. It's odd, though, that people are willing, even eager, to ask for seconds on just about everything except medical diagnoses. It is always a good idea, for your health as well as your pocketbook, to get a **second**

opinion on any invasive procedure your doctor recommends, whether diagnostic or surgical. Review the information on benefits in your insurance plan concerning when a second opinion is required and covered. Some companies require a second opinion for all elective procedures; however, if you forgo the second opinion, you may discover that your coverage has been reduced by half. But regardless of who pays, it is always smart to get a second opinion, especially if a trip to the hospital looms in your near future. Studies show that there is often substantial disagreement about diagnoses and treatment options.

◆ *Get more than two opinions when the*
 first two disagree.

If the second opinion does not agree with the first, it is often a good idea to get a third or even fourth opinion. What you are looking for is a consensus among practitioners, which allows you to make an informed decision about the best course of action. A thorough investigation on your part is the surest way to avoid unnecessary treatment and to save money in the long run.

◆ *Get independent second opinions.*
 Don't rely on a second-opinion referral
 from your own doctor.

A lot of second-opinion doctors recommended by first-opinion doctors turn out to be professional ditto marks and not all that valuable in terms of independent judgments. This is true in part because surgeons are the doctors most often asked for second opinions, and they're hardly predisposed to recommend sheathing the knife. It's also true that doctors often refer patients to other doctors for nonmedical reasons, such as the fact that they're golf buddies or "I owe him a favor." You are less likely to get an impartial, objective second opinion from your doctor's friend or close colleague. In addition, chances are that your doctor will call and discuss your case with the person to whom he referred you, and the second opinion will be made before the second doctor has a chance to examine you.

To find your own physician for a second opinion, start by contacting your insurance company and requesting a list of physicians who participate in second-opinion programs. Do the same with your employer's benefits manager and your union, if you're a union member. Check the *Directory of Medical Specialists* in your local library's reference section. Ask friends who might have had similar conditions what doctor they used. The point is, shop around to find the most objective and competent practitioner available.

◆ *Explore non-M.D. providers when possible.*

Basic health care can often be provided competently, safely and less expensively by non-M.D.'s such as **optometrists, podiatrists, chiropractors, audiologists, physician assistants, nurse-midwives** and **nurse practitioners**. A quick glance through the medical-services section of the *Dictionary of Occupational Titles* will find hundreds of professional occupations concerned with treating and caring for sick and injured people. Some of these practitioners support and complement the services of doctors and dentists, while others practice independently, depending upon the laws of the particular states in which they are licensed.

These so-called limited license providers can save you money if used properly. As a savvy consumer, you should always check their credentials to make certain they are properly licensed or certified—especially if your insurance plan requires that all non-M.D. providers be licensed or certified in accordance with the laws of your state.

Check, too, with your managed-care company to find out what type of practitioners' services are covered. Recently, some HMOs have been covering alternative and complementary therapies on a limited basis. These include naturopaths, homeopaths and others.

◆ Call ahead to see if the doctor is running on time.

Just as the savvy traveler calls the airport to see if a flight is on schedule, you can save a lot of time (and money if you must take time off from work) if you call your doctor's office and ask whether appointments are running on schedule. And if you see a doctor regularly, ask the receptionist to call *you* if appointments are running late. This allows you to either adjust your schedule or change the appointment.

◆ Send the doctor a bill if she keeps you waiting for more than 30 minutes.

The idea that patients actually bill doctors for waiting time is no longer a novelty. (Not long ago, a savvy Florida man sued his doctor for excessive waiting and won!) Medical practice management experts have taken note of this and are now telling doctors that they had better get used to it. One expert told a doctor to adjust the patient's bill for the next office visit. In short, value your time and remember that if you end up not seeing the doctor, you have lost not only the time in the waiting room, but also the time it took you to get there and back.

◆ Use a doctor with separate waiting rooms for sick and well visits.

More and more doctors are offering this convenience, particularly for children. Doctors' offices are prime places to pick up illnesses, and more illnesses mean more money. How smart is it to pay to see a doctor, then pay again for something you "caught" in the waiting room? If your doctor doesn't provide such a service, recommend that he do so.

◆ *Make sure the doctor accepts your insurance coverage.*

Always confirm, at the time you make the appointment, that the doctor accepts the health insurance that you carry *and* will accept your insurance reimbursement as "payment in full," less required copayments or **deductibles**. These three little words can lead to trouble if you and your doctor's billing staff are using the same words but speaking a different language. A simple misunderstanding here can lead to **balance billing**, the practice of billing the patient for the difference between the doctor's usual charge and the amount paid by the insurance company. Clarify these points ahead of time.

◆ *Get a job in a hospital.*

It may sound facetious, but it really can be a money saver. Hospitals often give employees free services—although in recent years, some hospitals have modified their benefits plans to include deductibles.

◆ *Make sure a family member becomes a doctor.*

But don't pay for the relative's education!

◆ *Don't offhandedly substitute an emergency room for your doctor.*

Never go to an ER (except in absolute emergencies) unless you at least try to contact your doctor first. If your doctor does not make provisions for seeing people at relatively short notice during office hours, find another doctor. To avoid out-of-pocket expenses, check your insurance coverage concerning when ER visits are covered and when not. Another reason for avoiding the ER, if possible, is what you may encounter there—less than desirable conditions and possibly a long wait. Some reports indicate that a wait of seven to 10 hours is not that unusual in certain cities and regions; so such a visit not only costs you more money, but it also wastes your valuable time.

If you are enrolled in an HMO, ideally your HMO will want you to use its emergency center or an affiliated hospital's ER for immediate treatment. However, as you know, not every emergency situation is so strategically and conveniently orchestrated. Find out your HMO's rules in the event you seek emergency care during night or weekend hours or when away from home, as well as its rule should your calls to your primary-care physician go unanswered. Be smart and find out *ahead* of the time you *really* need this information.

◆ *Seek telephone advice from your doctor whenever possible.*

Most doctors are happy to answer questions and provide advice over the phone about medication, reactions to treatment or recurring health problems. Ever since the People's Medical Society promoted the use of set-aside telephone hours in our physician Code of Practice (see pages 21 and 22), the concept has been catching on. You can save a considerable amount of money and perhaps unnecessary anguish by avoiding office visits for simple medical advice.

◆ *Get to know your doctor's office staff.*

Many problems can be solved and questions answered by a doctor's office staff, and, frankly, it's just smart to make yourself known to the people who control really important aspects of a medical practice. Patients are generally not charged for brief consultations with the office nurse—by phone or in person.

◆ *Demand that the doctor accept Medicare payments on assignment.*

Most doctors are willing to accept Medicare on **assignment**—which means that you will not be required to pay more than your 20 percent copayment—on a case-by-case basis. If your doctor is hesitant about accepting assignment, remind her that most doctors do accept it and that you would consider switching physicians over the issue. If your doctor refuses, find another doctor.

If you can't find another doctor or don't want to switch, you should know that there is a limit to the amount of balance billing that she may do. This means that **nonpartici-pating physicians**—physicians that don't accept assignment— may charge you no more than 115 percent of the Medicare-approved amount and not the full difference between their regular fee and the Medicare-approved amount.

◆ *Read about your condition.*

You will be able to make savvy, more informed decisions about your treatment—and avoid possibly unnecessary tests and procedures—if you know a lot about your condition and ask logical and informed questions. Only then will you be able to be a major partner in making your health decisions. And don't neglect to take advantage of a free service right there in your own community: your local public library. If you have not discovered the resources, ingenuity and help-fulness that a reference librarian has to offer, then by all means, do so. Even if you live in a small community with a modest library, one with a limited catalog of medical and health books, there's always interlibrary loan. In addition, hospitals will often let you use their medical libraries.

If you have access to a computer with a modem, get on the information superhighway. Indeed, the Internet is loaded with excellent medical and health sites. And there are many health chat groups on the Internet that allow you to speak to others about your condition. A word of caution, however, about cyberspace health: Be careful of the sources of in-formation. Since the Internet is essentially a large bulletin board without supervision, anybody can put any kind of information on it. That means it is up to you to determine if the information you read is valid, sound and worthy of your consideration.

◆ *Say no if you do not understand, and*
ask questions until you do.

Never submit to a test, treatment or procedure that you
do not fully understand. You should be able to answer four
questions about any treatment your doctor recommends:

1. What is the purpose of this test/procedure/medication?
2. How will it help my condition?
3. Are there less costly, and equally safe, alternatives to
   what is proposed?
4. What are the possible **side effects**, and what is the
   probability that one or more will occur?

Don't be intimidated by comments such as "Who's the
doctor here?" or "It's to make you better." Every unnecessary
test or procedure costs you money, not to mention time and
possible discomfort.

◆ *Demand a full justification of any tests*
or procedures.

Just as noted above, you can make an informed decision
about your doctor's recommendations only if you understand
them and you know why a particular treatment is preferable
to others.

◆ *Look for free or low-priced community services.*

Many communities offer flu shots, immunizations, simple
screening tests, cholesterol screening, occult blood screening
and certain other health-related services through the county
health department. Also, visit health fairs in your area to
learn more about services that are available in your community at no or nominal cost.

◆ *Always ask if it is possible to use previous x-rays rather than take new ones.*

Doctors often order x-rays because they do not know that previous x-rays exist. Keep a complete record of x-rays—what type, when, how many different exposures—and request that x-rays be promptly sent to a new doctor. Even simple x-rays are expensive (and can be dangerous), so they should be taken only if absolutely necessary.

◆ *Avoid mobile x-ray units.*

Mobile x-ray units often use miniature films that require a greater x-ray exposure. Also, these mobile units are used primarily for chest screening for tuberculosis, which is usually unnecessary.

◆ *If you are a woman under 50, consult your physician about the need for routine mammography.*

In light of recent headlines on breast cancer rates, the savvy medical consumer who's a woman undoubtedly is wondering what to do and when. There is great debate among medical experts about when it is useful to begin routine mammography. The benefits of mammography for women between the ages of 50 and 74 seem to be clear. As reported in the January 11, 1995, issue of the *Journal of the American Medical Association,* a meta-analysis of 13 studies that examined mammography screening and breast cancer death rates among women aged 40 to 49 and aged 50 to 74 found the following:

▶ There was a significant reduction in breast cancer deaths in women aged 50 to 74 who underwent regular screening (at 18- to 33-month intervals).

▶ The reduction in the death rates from breast cancer among women aged 50 and older ranged from 20 to 39 percent.

▶ The studies did not discover a reduction in breast cancer mortality in women younger than 50 who underwent screening mammography for seven to nine years.

Since some women under the age of 50 may be at a higher breast cancer risk than the general population, the American College of Physicians recommends that women between the ages of 40 and 49 discuss their personal situations with their doctors concerning mammography. This recommendation is shared by the American Academy of Family Physicians, the U.S. Preventive Task Force and the National Women's Health Network.

However, the National Cancer Institute, the American Cancer Society, the American College of Gynecologists and Obstetricians, Planned Parenthood Federation of America and 20 other groups support routine screening for all women aged 40 and older.

You should also remember that insurance companies usually will not reimburse for diagnostic tests that aren't medically necessary. This means that any such expense comes out of your pocket. In any case, be sure to discuss mammography thoroughly with your doctor.

◆ *Avoid fluoroscopy if an ordinary x-ray can do the job.*

Fluoroscopy exposes you to much more x-ray radiation and, therefore, should never be used if a simple x-ray will serve. Overkill on tests is a tendency many doctors have— and it's your wallet (and health) that suffers.

◆ *Question routine preemployment x-rays.*

People whose jobs will require them to handle food or work with people are often required to be screened for tuberculosis by state laws. Nowadays, there are perfectly acceptable non-x-ray tests to screen for tuberculosis that do not require radiation, so resist a chest x-ray for this purpose.

◆ *Refuse routine dental x-rays.*

Again, x-ray examinations are expensive and possibly dangerous, so you should never agree to them unless they are necessary to diagnose a problem.

◆ *If you change dentists or go to a dental specialist, take your dental x-rays with you.*

There is no reason to submit to an additional set of x-rays by a new dentist if you have had x-rays done recently. Just take your old ones along with you.

◆ *If you've had three or more normal Pap smears one year apart, ask your doctor if the Pap test may be performed less frequently.*

In 1988, the American Cancer Society adopted this policy, similar to that endorsed by the American College of Obstetricians and Gynecologists, the National Cancer Institute and the American Medical Association. What's a good time interval? A recent study by researchers at the University of Washington in Seattle suggests that going more than two years without a Pap smear increases your risk of developing cervical cancer.

◆ *Have routine screening tests done by non-M.D.'s.*

In many cases, routine screening tests can be done just as accurately by non-M.D.'s—for example, nurse-midwives in the case of Pap smears. It is usually more expensive to take the time of a fully qualified physician to perform simple tests than to use a nurse or other non-M.D.

◆ *Keep your own medical record.*

Although medical information technology is improving and medical record keeping is moving out of the dark ages into computers, it is a savvy medical consumer who keeps her own medical record. In the modern medical age, most people see many doctors over the course of a lifetime. As a result, your complete medical history resides in no one place. There are any number of ways to keep track of your medical record, from a file drawer to books on the subject. We recommend *Your Complete Medical Record* (Allentown, PA: People's Medical Society, 1993).

By knowing when you had a particular illness, what medications you were allergic to or when you were hospitalized (and what happened while you were), you will be able to assist future medical practitioners in serving you.

◆ *Seek out the best medical advice.*

Seek out the best medical advice you can get, especially if your doctor is having trouble making a diagnosis or recommends invasive surgery or an "exotic" or risky treatment. Don't be lulled into thinking your doctor, or even any doctor in your community, knows the right answer.

When in doubt, contact a major medical school or one of America's best teaching hospitals (usually located in major cities). Ask for the chairperson of the department that is associated with your problem. Tell him what the problem is and what has happened so far. Ask if the situation sounds right to him. Also, ask for a recommendation to an expert who might be close to you. You'll be surprised at how easy it is to contact these individuals, and you'll feel much more satisfied knowing you have gone to the best for advice.

◆ *Take a family member or friend into the examining room with you.*

Most of us are nervous, even afraid, when it comes to going to the doctor. This is particularly true if we are sick or worried about what the doctor might find. Therefore, it's good policy to always take a family member or friend into the examining room with you. Why? Well, the most important reason is to have another set of ears. Often in our nervousness, we miss what the doctor is saying. Another set of ears will help to verify what the doctor has said. Also, a family member or friend can ask questions you are too upset to ask.

If your doctor or his nurse gives you a hard time about bringing someone into the room with you, explain that you need the assistance the other person provides. And if your doctor absolutely forbids it, find another doctor.

◆ *Take a tape recorder to your doctor's office.*

When you can't take a family member or friend with you to the doctor, take a tape recorder along. The idea is not to catch your doctor in a lie or to have a record for a malpractice suit, but rather to make sure you heard and understood everything the doctor said. Was that two pills four times a day or four pills two times a day? Having a tape recorder with you allows you to play back what the doctor said at your own leisure, when you're more relaxed and when you can give it your undivided attention.

◆ *Bring a list of questions to ask your doctor.*

Think before you go to the doctor. Make a list of all the questions you want to ask the doctor once you are there. Don't be afraid to pull out the list and fire away once you have his attention. Studies show that the average doctor allows the patient 18 seconds of talking time before he interrupts. If you have a list of questions with you, you won't be easily distracted. If your doctor seems agitated about your questions or the fact that you have a list, explain how important it is that you understand what is going on. Also note that, ultimately, you must make your own medical decisions, and the only way that can be done is with information.

Drugs

You don't need to be an economist to know that the cost of prescription drugs has gone through the roof. In the 1980s, the overall inflation rate was 58 percent, while drug prices increased a whopping 152 percent. In the early 1990s, it was a different story, as the inflation rate fell from 7.8 percent to around 3.7 percent by mid-decade. However, this did not necessarily mean consumers were given a price break.

What is a bitter pill for you, the consumer, to swallow is a prescription for profit for the drug manufacturing industry. A 1995 report by Families USA, a Washington-based public interest group, revealed that the profit rate for the manufacturers of the 20 top-selling prescription drugs was five times higher than the median profit rate for all Fortune 500 companies—15 percent versus 3 percent.

How can you stay on the winning side in this multibillion-dollar-a-year industry? Think smart and know where to go to find out whether the drug your doctor prescribes for you is the best, most effective medication for your condition. Granted, in a nation that fills approximately 2.3 billion prescriptions each year and has some 2,500 drugs on the market, even the wisest of medical consumers cannot become familiar with the names of all the available prescription and **over-the-counter (OTC) drugs**. But arm yourself with information on as many "fronts" as you can: everything from choosing the best pharmacist and comparison-shopping for OTC, brand-name and **generic drugs** to avoiding costly and potentially dangerous medication errors.

◆ *Know your pharmacist.*

A pharmacist can be an invaluable resource for information regarding drugs—any **interactions** to be aware of, alternative forms of the same drug (i.e., liquid or pill) and less expensive alternatives. The pharmacist is the most readily accessible health-care professional most of us have—a highly trained drug expert who probably knows more than your own physician about the relative benefits and risks of various drugs. With the greater complexity of today's medications and, in some cases, the greater potency, the savvy medical consumer will find a competent and communicative pharmacist. It's also smart to talk with your pharmacist, for the better she knows you, the more she will be able to help.

◆ *Shop around for prescription prices.*

Prescription drug prices vary about as much as a nervous stock market, and it's no secret that most prescription medications go up in cost every year. So now, more than ever, you have got to find better prices for the medications you need. Contact the large chain pharmacies in your area first since they usually offer better discounts because of their bulk-buying practices. Also, consider nontraditional prescription drug outlets such as Wal-Mart or K-Mart. Often, they use their pharmacy departments as loss leaders, selling certain prescriptions below wholesale cost as a way to lure you into the store. And even if you have an insured prescription plan where you work, shopping for the lowest drug price is important, especially if you have a copayment based on a percentage of the total cost.

WHAT A GOOD PHARMACIST DOES:
A CHECKLIST

✔ Reads doctors' prescriptions, fills them, labels them and charges appropriately.

✔ Keeps important family medication records, called patient medication profiles, and uses them to prevent allergic reactions to drugs, dangerous interactions, duplicate medications and drug abuse.

✔ Advises, both in person and in writing, how to use prescription and nonprescription medication; how and when to take it; what the possible side effects are; what the shelf life is; how to store the medication; and whether there is potential for dangerous interactions with foods and/or other medications.

✔ Answers your questions about the staggering variety of medicines, remedies, tonics, pills, elixirs, lotions, salves, capsules and powders on the market.

✔ Advises you, when necessary, to seek a medical practitioner's help.

◆ Buy generic prescription drugs.

A generic drug (the name of which is usually a condensed version of the drug's original chemical name) is one whose active ingredients duplicate those of the brand-name product. While a generic does not have to be the same size, shape or color of the brand name, by law it does have to be bioequivalent. A generic cannot differ from the pioneer drug by more than 20 percent in either the speed or amount of absorption.

On the average, generic drugs are 30 percent cheaper than their brand-name cousins—even 50 to 70 percent cheaper than the more expensive medicines. Mind you, the generic is *usually* cheaper than the brand-name drug, but always check with your doctor or pharmacist to determine whether a generic form of the drug you need is available, safe and less expensive. Also, since laws vary across the country, ask what your state's law is concerning the substitution of generic for brand-name drugs. For more information about generic drugs in general or specific generic products, talk to your pharmacist.

◆ *Buy store-brand over-the-counter drugs.*

Many pharmacies and some grocery store chains purchase OTC drugs in bulk and package them under their own store's brand name or label. Compare prices of brand-name items with those of the less expensive, but identical, store-brand items.

---

10 OF THE MOST COMMONLY PRESCRIBED DRUGS AND THEIR GENERIC VERSIONS

Brand Name/Generic Name	Usage
Amoxil/amoxicillin	antibiotic
Keflex/cephalexin	antibiotic
Lanoxin/digoxin	heart
Lasix/furosemide	diuretic
Premarin/conjugated estrogen	hormone replacement
Procardia XL/nifedipine	high blood pressure, angina
Synthroid/levothyroxine	thyroid hormone
Trimox/amoxicillin	antibiotic
Tylenol 3/acetaminophen with codeine	pain relief
Xanax/alprazolam	tranquilizer

But before you plunk down your cash for an OTC remedy with possibly questionable effectiveness, find out if a formerly prescription-only drug is available without a prescription. As the Food and Drug Administration (FDA) lifted the prescription-only restriction from many products (most notably **decongestants**, antacids and hydrocortisone), OTC medications became available to treat the same symptoms that prescription drugs treated. The effectiveness of these medications has been proven, and it makes sense to spend your money on these products.

Indeed, Americans treat their ailments without professional help and with nonprescription medicines some 60 percent of the time, according to *American Pharmacy* magazine. Before you self-medicate, however, talk with your doctor or pharmacist about similar OTC drugs. As for the FDA's stamp of approval or its eagerness to remove a suspect drug from the market, let's just say that ineffective and marginally effective drugs do exist.

A word of warning, though: The savvy medical consumer makes a point of consulting a pharmacist or physician before buying any OTC preparations for babies, young children, the elderly, debilitated persons or pregnant or breast-feeding women.

◆ *Buy single-ingredient OTC drugs.*

Many OTC drugs are preparations containing several drugs—for example, a cold medication that combines an **antihistamine** with a decongestant. It is less expensive to purchase a decongestant and an antihistamine separately because often you will need only one of these to treat your symptoms and because mixtures can be more expensive.

Here are a few other wise strategies for selecting the best OTC drugs and getting the most for your money:

▶ Find out the risks or side effects of any OTC drugs you're considering buying and taking.

▶ Ask about potentially dangerous interactions between OTC medications and any prescription drugs you may be taking. Common products such as nose drops, antacids and aspirin can interfere with prescription drugs.

▶ Go over with your pharmacist the label instructions of any medication so that you can be sure you're taking it wisely and appropriately, especially if you're taking drug preparations in forms you do not normally use or fully understand— suppositories or prolonged-release tablets, for instance.

◆ Break the code.

What we are talking about is the shorthand code that doctors, pharmacists and nurses share as part of a long tradition of cryptic communication that excludes consumers. Particularly prominent are the medical abbreviations that are scrawled across prescription forms. Here's a list of some Latin directions to pharmacists and abbreviations that turn up frequently on prescription sheets (some doctors may use variations of these symbols):

Abbreviation (on Prescription)	English Meaning
ad lib.	as needed
a.c.	before meals
p.c.	after meals
b.i.d.	twice a day
t.i.d.	three times a day
q.i.d.	four times a day
h.s.	at bedtime
p.o.	orally (by mouth)
q.4h	every four hours
q.8h	every eight hours
ut dict.	as directed by doctor
OD	right eye (drops)
OS	left eye (drops)
OU	both eyes (drops)

◆ *Ask for an initial one- to two-day supply of any new prescription to check for side effects.*

Since the possibility exists for an **adverse reaction** to *any* medication, you will save your health and money if you initially request only a one- to two-day supply of a new prescription. You can pick up the remainder of the prescription (and pay for it) the next day if no adverse reaction occurs.

◆ *Ask your doctor for free samples.*

Physicians regularly receive free samples of prescription and OTC medications from pharmaceutical company representatives. Think of it as a test drive, something any savvy consumer would do first.

◆ *Purchase drugs directly from your doctor.*

Let us first say that the practice called physician dispensing is not without its critics; indeed, the entire issue has raised quite a hue and cry in the prescription drug industry— in part because it upsets the so-called natural order of business wherein doctors prescribe and pharmacists dispense. The pharmacists call it an encroachment on their territory and a source of potential harm to consumers. Meanwhile, the doctors call it good for their patients and bottom-line smart for their incomes.

What has made this a growth industry is a relatively new business called **repackaging**: Companies (called repackagers) buy drugs in bulk at wholesale costs from drug manufacturers, then resell to doctors in convenient, safety-sealed containers, ready for on-the-spot dispensing to their patients.

The savvy medical consumer will get all the facts before buying and taking any prescription drug dispensed by her physician:

▶ Compare the doctor's prices with those of area drugstores to determine whether there is an economic advantage.

▶ Verify if anyone in the doctor's office assures that the

drugs dispensed are the right ones, the dosages correct and the directions clear, complete and accurate. (After all, physician dispensing sidesteps the highly trained drug expert, the pharmacist.)

▶ If you have insurance that pays for all or part of your prescription medication, make sure it will pay for medication bought directly from your practitioner.

◆ *Purchase in bulk, when appropriate.*

Although individuals cannot buy drugs directly from wholesalers, bulk purchasing is a way you can purchase your medications in larger quantities. If you're taking a certain medication for an extended period of time, have your physician write the prescription for a six-month or longer supply, as opposed to six refills. Some pharmacists may be wary if you ask for your six refills all at once, and your state's pharmacy laws may prohibit such dispensing. If you have your physician write in the number of pills—such as 200 or 250—then you can discuss bulk purchases with the pharmacist. And don't be afraid to negotiate the price of a bulk purchase. When you buy larger quantities of a medication, it means less time and money spent by the pharmacy filling your prescription. Some of that savings should be passed along directly to you. Negotiation is easier with a small or locally owned pharmacy where the owner/pharmacist can make a price deal with you. Large local or national chains generally do not have anyone in a position to bargain with you at the local store.

◆ *Investigate purchasing by mail order.*

The cost savings of doing such, according to the industry's trade organization, range anywhere from 5 to 40 percent off the prices at your local pharmacy. Most prescription drug insurance programs offered through employers have a mail-order component as part of the service. The American Association of Retired Persons (and other trade and social groups) offers a full-service mail-order pharmacy to members. Other mail-order businesses offer more specialized medications such as **homeopathic remedies** and vitamin and mineral supplements. Before you buy by mail, compare prices with several local pharmacies to be sure you are saving money.

◆ *Ask about any available discount.*

Many, if not most, pharmacies offer senior citizen discounts. Infants' and children's discounts are also available in some pharmacies. Ask the pharmacist for details.

◆ *Purchase or use a prescription plan.*

In recent years, the number of prescription drug insurance plans has grown dramatically. Most large employers now provide them to their employees. Many smaller employers have them as well. And you do not have to be employed to take advantage of these programs. The federal government even approves and regulates such programs for certain types of Medicare supplemental insurance, also called Medigap, policies. Check out these policies with an insurer that sells Medigap insurance in your state.

Generally, prescription drug programs issue you a card. You take your prescription and the card to a pharmacy accepting your drug program and get your prescription filled. You usually must pay a small copayment, usually $5 to $10 per prescription, and the rest is billed to the insurer. If your prescription costs less than the copayment, you pay the lower of the two prices.

Even if you do not have a program like the one above, you may have coverage for prescription medication under your health insurance plan. Most traditional **fee-for-service** and **indemnity insurance plans** that offer major medical coverage provide for some noninpatient medications. Usually, you must first pay an annual out-of-pocket deductible, anywhere from $100 to $500, after which the insurer starts paying up to 80 percent or more of your prescription drug costs.

◆ *Keep a patient medication profile on yourself (or make sure someone else is doing so).*

No doubt about it—someone should be keeping a medication profile on you and on everyone else in your household. It's a system that monitors all the drugs you are taking, in hopes of avoiding medication errors. Actually, the logical site for the profile is your pharmacy. The American Pharmaceutical Association recommends that a patient medication profile contain the following information:

▶ Your name, address and phone number

▶ Your birthday, so that the pharmacist can check whether the dosage is age-appropriate

▶ Any allergies, reactions or adverse effects you've had

▶ A concise health history, including any conditions or diseases that would preclude the use of certain drugs

▶ The OTC medicines you take

▶ The date and number of each prescription filled for you, the name of the drug, its dosage and strength, quantity, directions for use and price

▶ The prescriber and dispenser of every medication you take

◆ *Properly store drugs.*

Most drug items need to be kept fresh, just as many food products do, with cool, dry conditions best for preserving them. True, some people, especially those who might in an emergency need to get to their medications at a moment's notice, like to keep multiple vials of their prescription drugs stashed away—in the workshop or even in the car. But tossing pills in with the maps and owner's manual is a prescription for trouble—and meltdown. Ask your pharmacist how to store the drugs you are purchasing.

◆ *Guard against overmedication.*

It's a fact that drug overdosing occurs in many hospitals' pediatric wards and nurseries. The dosages—some as much as 10 times greater than prescribed—are the result of misplaced decimal points and sloppy computational skills of nurses and doctors who do not understand the appropriate doses for different age groups. But that's not all. Various reports have pointed out that drug overdosing occurs with the low-weight elderly. Not only are doctors failing to adjust doses for body weight in many cases, but they often also are not taking into account the ages of the patients. The operative physiological fact here is that the older you get, the longer it takes for drugs to clear out of your system, so dosages must be adjusted accordingly.

It just makes sense, doesn't it, that correct dosages vary among people just as their ages and weights vary? If a savvy medical consumer knows this, shouldn't a doctor? Well, the problem, according to one study, is that doctors prescribe "by habit, with little adjustment for individual patients." So the next time your doctor writes a prescription for you, ask her to double-check your weight and age against the recommended standard dosage for that medication. It may mean a double-savvy whammy: You'll save money if the effective drug dose is less, and you'll increase your margin of safety for dose-related side effects.

◆ *Purchase drugs from your HMO pharmacy.*

If you are a member of an HMO, find out if it has an in-house pharmacy. HMO pharmacies often sell drugs to members at wholesale cost or slightly above.

◆ *Consult drug reference books.*

To learn more about the medications that are prescribed for you and your family, consult a drug reference guide. You'll find them in libraries as well as pharmacies. A good guide will list the medication by class—such as an antidiabetic or a calcium channel blocker—by chemical or generic name and by brand name. There should also be a section in which the medication is described and the condition(s) given for which the medication may be prescribed. Additional sections usually discuss how to use the medication, when not to use it in conjunction with other medications and what the side effects and **contraindications** (reasons you shouldn't use the medication) are.

Two good reference guides are the ***Physician's Desk Reference (PDR)*** and *The Complete Drug Reference,* the latter published by Consumer Reports Books. Clearly, the best time to find out that a drug may not be appropriate for you is before you have gone to the expense of having the prescription filled.

◆ *Consult consumer buying guides to drugs.*

Buying guides to drugs, written especially for consumers, are available in most libraries. In addition to giving you information about specific medications, they also point out which drugs are the most effective and which drugs are not effective. Using the most effective drug for a given condition is ultimately cheaper. Here are some guides you may want to look for:

The Complete Drug Reference. (Yonkers, N.Y.: Consumer Reports Books, 1996).

Everything You Need to Know About Drugs. (Springhouse, Pa.: Springhouse Corp., 1996).

The People's Guide to Deadly Drug Interactions. Teresa Graedon, Ph.D., and Joe Graedon. (New York: St. Martin's Press, 1995).

The PDR Family Guide to Prescription Drugs 3d ed. (Montvale, N.J.: Medical Economics Data, 1995).

Worst Pills, Best Pills II. Sidney Wolfe, M.D., et al. (Washington, D.C.: Public Citizen Health Research Group, 1993).

Hospitals

Where you get your medical care is as important as who provides it. The setting not only dictates what treatment you get or do not get, but also how much you pay.

You don't have to be a cost accountant to realize that certain health-care settings are more expensive than others, with hospital-based care the steepest. One night in a hospital costs between $380 and $500; an average stay costs a total of $3,080 (March 1994 figures). And that covers only the room and meals; when drugs, medical tests and other charges are factored in, the daily cost climbs sharply to between $880 and $1,500. In terms of national impact, the dollars and cents quickly add up. In 1995, $365 billion was spent for hospital care. That amounts to $1,400 for every man, woman and child in the country.

Dollar figures like these are enough to convince most people to reduce the time spent in the hospital, if not completely eliminate hospitalization in favor of another setting. But if you must go in, pay close attention to procedures and medications ordered by your physician, and make sure you know what has been ordered and that you are fully informed of the whys and wherefores. Further, if you must go in, it stands to reason that a close scrutiny of the entire process, from preadmission talks with your doctor to admission and on to discharge, has the potential to save you money and gets you intimately involved in important decisions about your health and welfare.

Speak up whenever you find something is not what you have been told. Be on the lookout for errors in medications, procedures and the like that can end up costing you extra days in the hospital, as well as extra money from your pocket.

Using even one of the following money-saving hints will save you *at least* the price of this book. And that's just savvy personal finance!

◆ Don't go unless absolutely necessary.

An unnecessary stay threatens far more than your wallet, as if money alone weren't enough to make you quibble over the necessity of hospitalization. Hospitals can be hazardous to your health. While in the hospital, not only are you at risk of piling up mounds of charges for procedures and tests, but you are also at risk of acquiring a condition you did not have when you went in. That happens to one out of every five hospital patients, and these conditions not only require additional treatment at additional cost, but they can be deadly as well. One of these so-called iatrogenic (literally, doctor-produced) conditions—**nosocomial infection**—is produced by microorganisms that dwell with relative impunity in hospitals. Most develop at least 72 hours after admission, which means that some may not become manifest until after discharge.

You could describe nosocomial infections as expensive souvenirs of your hospital stay. And close to one out of every 10 patients admitted to a hospital acquires one of these nasty, and often preventable, souvenirs. It is estimated that the recovery time necessary to combat a nosocomial infection is about four extra days of stay. Expensive as they are—experts estimate that they add, at a minimum, $2.5 billion to America's annual medical bill—nosocomial infections can also be deadly souvenirs: Some tallies of infection-related deaths run as high as 100,000 (other estimates are even higher—300,000 or so) a year. The Centers for Disease Control and Prevention estimates that 80,000 hospital deaths a year are attributable to nosocomial infections.

What does the savvy medical consumer do, however, who needs a particular medical procedure? If you require a surgical procedure, you may be able to avoid the hospital entirely if the surgery can be done on an outpatient basis (see page 56). Ask your physician about this option. Outpatient surgery is usually less expensive than inpatient surgery, and you lessen the risk of picking up a nasty germ while in the hospital. In fact, your insurance plan or your employer may require you to investigate outpatient surgery first.

There's also the matter of copayment, that cost-sharing requirement in many insurance policies in which you assume a portion or percentage of the cost of covered services. If your copayment is 20 percent on inpatient services and only 10 percent on outpatient services—a not unlikely scenario—it's to your advantage to select the outpatient setting.

◆ *Make sure hospital personnel wash their hands before touching you.*

Of all the potentially protective measures you can take (or insist that your caregivers take), this one merits its own individual mention. Why? Well, because most of the hospital-acquired infections are gotten from the contaminated hands of doctors, nurses and other hospital personnel. The Institute for Child Health Policy and others report that many hospital workers who come in direct contact with patients don't take the time, or are not concerned enough, to perform the simplest and best known of precautionary actions. And doctors are among the worst offenders. You can greatly lower your chances of catching such an infection—and paying for its treatment—simply by refusing to allow hospital personnel to care for you until they have washed their hands.

◆ *Protect yourself from nosocomial infections.*

There is no surefire defense for you if the rest of the hospital is a vast and bubbling breeding ground. So the first step is to try to gain admission to a hospital that has a good (meaning low) nosocomial infection record. Ask your doctor about it. Contact your local department of health. Ask the hospital directly, but be on your guard if the hospital paints too rosy a picture. That may mean that the staff is not properly surveying the facility's infection rate, or not surveying it at all. Ask to speak to the infection officer at the hospital. (If it doesn't have one, don't check in!)

The other line of defense is to be informed. Remember that a savvy medical consumer is armed with information. Know the work areas of the hospital where you are at higher risk:

▶ *Hemodialysis unit.* The equipment here can be a source of hepatitis B, a virulent organism that is difficult to destroy.

▶ *Infant nursery.*

▶ *Intensive care unit.* Usually occupied by patients who are extremely weak and thus susceptible to infection, this unit is operated under emergency measures that often have to forsake pristine sanitary procedures in order to save a life.

▶ *Operating room.*

Nosocomial infections can also pass to patients via the procedural chain of the food services department, due to any one or more factors—nearly all of them with their roots in human error. Studies also point to other work areas in the hospital that, because of persistently poor and unprofessional hygiene practices, are breeding grounds, too: the central service department (the unit responsible for processing, storing and dispensing hospital supplies); the pharmacy; the laundry; and the laboratory (where, more than one story goes, workers have to be admonished not to keep their lunches in the same refrigerators as the ones that contain serum or other specimens).

◆ *Assert yourself.*

While it is true that one-third of all infections treated in hospitals are nosocomial infections, it is also estimated that as many as half are preventable. The savvy medical consumer is, where necessary, assertive. Here are some actions you can take while in the hospital:

▶ If your roommate becomes infected or if you are concerned that what he has could possibly be transmitted to you via the air or through the use of a common bathroom, ask your doctor or the staff nurse-epidemiologist about your risks. Change your room at once if there is any chance you might become infected, because once you are infected, it is too late.

▶ If you are undergoing surgery or a procedure that requires the removal of hair, refuse to be shaven the night before surgery. One study indicates that among people shaved the day prior to their operations, the nosocomial infection rate is 5.6 percent. Chemical depilatories reduce the rate to just 0.6 percent. Using barber clippers to remove hair the morning of surgery yields a low infection rate, too.

▶ Question whether shaving or clipping is necessary at all. Maybe not—and especially when it comes to ob-gyn situations. Removing hair before vaginal delivery or surgery in that area is probably uncalled for, because the old idea that hair creates a climate for infection is unsubstantiated by clinical studies.

▶ Have nurses regularly check the drainage of urinary catheters to help maintain cleanliness.

◆ *If you deliver your baby in the hospital, get her out of there as soon as possible.*

Sure, you've heard that new mothers and their babies are being kicked out of hospitals in less than a day. And you've read that any number of states and the federal government have passed laws assuring mothers-to-be that they will get at least two days in the hospital for uncomplicated childbirth and up to five days for **cesarean section (c-section)** deliveries. But don't fall victim to the hysteria. A woman and her baby should only stay in the hospital as long as is necessary to ensure health. And studies show that amount of time is very short, a day or so in most cases.

Birthing in hospitals exposes infants to the full range of hospital-acquired infections to which adults are exposed. Upper-respiratory and staph infections are common in hospital nurseries. And aside from the worry you will expend, you are required to pay for the necessary care to treat these infections. So the sooner that mother and child leave the hospital, the less chance that either will acquire an unnecessary and expensive infection.

And remember that both doctors and hospitals are legally liable if they force you or your baby to leave before either one of you is medically ready. Remind them of this fact if you feel you're being rushed out the door.

◆ *Refuse admission tests that are not pertinent to your illness or the reason for your hospitalization.*

Most hospitals routinely require a variety of blood and urine tests and an x-ray upon admission, whatever your age and physical health and whether or not you need them. The American College of Radiology has urged that chest x-rays be eliminated as a routine procedure for hospital admissions, tuberculosis screening and preemployment physicals, and as a general rule, it's good to avoid x-rays unless absolutely necessary because of the dangers associated with excessive radiation. It is in the best interest of your physical and financial health to refuse unnecessary routine testing.

◆ *Use outpatient services.*

Many invasive diagnostic tests and simple surgeries can be done on an outpatient basis, an arrangement whereby you arrive in the morning for the procedure and are back home again in the afternoon or evening. As an outpatient, you are not admitted to the hospital, but you receive hospital care (for example, laboratory work and x-rays) without occupying a hospital bed or without receiving room, board or general nursing care. The growth in outpatient care has been so phenomenal that more and more insurance companies are requiring that certain procedures be done on an outpatient basis—mainly because of the cost savings associated with that setting versus inpatient care. Make sure that you know the requirements and limitations of your insurance coverage; otherwise, you may end up paying substantial out-of-pocket costs. Remember that the less time you spend in the hospital, generally the cheaper it will be—and as we discussed before, the less likely you are to acquire a nosocomial infection.

But a word of caution about outpatient procedures: Outpatient facilities come in two forms—hospital owned and operated and privately owned (usually a physician or group of doctors own it). There may be a big difference in quality between the two. Hospital-owned facilities are usually viewed as part of the hospital, whether on the grounds or miles away. As such, when the hospital is inspected for licensure and accreditation, the outpatient program and facilities are also reviewed. Plus, the doctors affiliated with the outpatient program have gone through the hospital's review process, which carefully screens the doctor for competence and training.

This is not necessarily the case with privately owned outpatient facilities. Often, they are owned by a lone doctor who may or may not have an affiliation with a hospital. In addition, states inspect privately owned facilities for health and safety and little else. They tend not to be accredited by any organization. And while most insurance companies will pay your bill at one of these facilities, that in itself is no grounds to be reassured.

So buyer beware! There are many excellent privately owned outpatient facilities, and there are some less-than-wonderful hospital-owned outpatient programs. Look carefully before you say yes and ask a lot of questions.

◆ *Don't stay overnight for diagnostic tests.*

Most diagnostic tests can be done on an outpatient basis, in and out in one day. Again, if you don't have to spend a night in the hospital, don't do it. Remember that any stay in a hospital entails money *and* potential exposure to unwanted illness.

◆ *Go to the hospital that does the largest number of the procedure that you need.*

Studies have shown that you are less likely to suffer complications or die if you have your surgery or other invasive procedure done at a hospital that performs a large number (some experts recommend at least 200 per year) of such procedures. You save yourself a lot of money and untold amounts of suffering if you do what you can to assure the best outcome from the start. After all, you pay the price in more than dollars for their mistakes or inadequacies. To find out how often a particular procedure is done at a hospital, call and ask to speak with the medical director.

◆ *Avoid hospital price gouging.*

As recently as the early 1990s, we would have told you to avoid **for-profit** hospitals. Studies at the time found that they were 23 percent more expensive than their **nonprofit** counterparts. But today, that is not the case. In fact, with most hospitals less than half full (in 1995, only 45 percent of hospital beds were full on any given day), every hospital is in a cost-cutting struggle to stay open. That means you have to be especially careful about hospital price gouging.

It's not unusual to see a $2 pill you get at your local drugstore priced at $29 in the hospital. A toothbrush can cost as much as a defense department wrench. Even if you're fully insured and even if Medicare and Medicaid say they cover it all, the fact is that you will ultimately pay for this gouging in the form of increased premiums or higher copayments and deductibles.

But you can fight back. Make sure you get an itemized bill—one that lists *every single* charge. Review it carefully and challenge anything that doesn't look right. Bring your own medication to the hospital, particularly if you're already taking prescription drugs that will be continued while you are a patient. This will save you oodles of bucks. You may have to sign a release indicating that you brought your own medication and that the hospital is not liable for it. Sign it. You're an adult.

If you really feel that you are being gouged on a particular item or charge, and you are getting nowhere with the hospital people, contact your insurance company's fraud division. Let them know the issue and have them look into it. If you are on Medicare or Medicaid, contact your federal congressional representative. She is your Medicare/Medicaid insurance agent. Have her office look into the problem for you.

◆ *Check room rates in advance.*

Room rates vary from hospital to hospital. Again, the basic charge for a hospital room may range from $380 to $500 a day depending upon the type of hospital and region of the country. The cost of ancillary services (lab, supplies, nursing, etc.) can easily change that to $880 to $1,500 a day. If you have an insurance plan that pays only up to a certain amount, say $350 a day, you have to shop around for an affordable room.

◆ *Refuse to pay a hospital admitting fee or hospital release (or discharge) fee to your doctor.*

These fees, which are commonly charged by doctors for admitting you to and discharging you from the hospital, are unjustifiable on the basis of services rendered to you, the patient. Find out whether your doctor customarily charges such fees and discuss your objections prior to your admission to the hospital.

◆ *Negotiate a discounted fee with your doctor in exchange for allowing services from a resident.*

If you have no objection to having your surgery or other procedures performed by a resident physician, then make that clear to your doctor. Just remember, that is how residents *learn*. But make sure that you do not pay for more than you get.

◆ *Avoid c-section deliveries.*

One study has shown that more c-sections are performed at night and on weekends—partly because doctors want to get the delivery over with quickly and, therefore, are less willing to wait through a long labor.

C-section deliveries are major surgery. They are not only much more expensive than vaginal deliveries, but they also expose both mother and baby to additional risks. Further, studies show that only one out of four women who had a previous c-section delivery need have another one for the birth of a subsequent child. The adage "Once a cesarean, always a cesarean" is just not true. Indeed, the American College of Obstetricians and Gynecologists issued strong guidelines some years back stating that repeat cesarean deliveries should no longer be routine.

The best way to avoid a c-section delivery is to be as knowledgeable as you can about the birth process so that you will be better able to ask the right questions and evaluate your doctor's recommendations. Not all c-sections are avoidable, but a good many are—and with information on whys, wherefores and options, you can avoid unnecessary surgery.

◆ *Use a nurse-midwife or family practitioner as your birth attendant and consider alternative birth settings.*

At the outset, let us say that, clearly, where birth attendants and settings are concerned, different strokes for different folks. The savvy—and pregnant—medical consumer realizes that the type of childbirth experience she has depends very much on who she finds to deliver her baby and where she decides to have it.

There are two reasons you save money by choosing a practitioner other than an obstetrician as your birth attendant: Other birth attendants usually charge less in basic delivery fees, and they generally will not recommend a costly c-section or other expensive (and potentially dangerous) high-technology intervention unless it is absolutely necessary. For more information on nurse-midwife services, contact

> American College of Nurse-Midwives
> 818 Connecticut Ave., N.W., Suite 900
> Washington, DC 20005
> 202-728-9860

Developed by **midwives** believing it to be the best alternative to both hospital and home deliveries, the birth center ideally offers a home*like* environment, a relaxed, flexible atmosphere and very little intervention in the birth process. Birth centers are designed to provide maternity care to women judged to be at low risk of obstetric complications, and this approach enjoys a loyal following of doctors, midwives, childbirth educators and consumers who champion the low complication and c-section rates, safety, consumer satisfaction and cost savings that many birth centers offer. A 1994 survey showed that, for a normal birth, birth centers offer a 31 to 46 percent cost savings over hospitals, depending on the length of stay. For more information, contact

National Association of Childbearing Centers
3123 Gottschall Rd.
Perkiomenville, PA 18074
215-234-8068

There is also growing interest in home births, and if your insurance plan will cover such services, it's worthwhile to investigate your options. For more information, contact

National Association of Parents and Professionals
    for Safe Alternatives in Childbirth
Route 1, Box 646
Marble Hill, MO 63764
573-238-2010

◆ *Become acquainted with the hospital's birthing policies and routine services before choosing to deliver there.*

From a cost perspective, you should be looking for hospital policies that encourage rooming-in (keeping the baby in the room with you) and early discharge (generally after 24 hours rather than two days [see our earlier discussion on page 55]). Often, hospitals charge for routine birth services—such as enemas, IVs and use of the delivery room—that not every woman receives. Scrutinize the bill and don't pay for any service you didn't receive. (And don't permit your insurance company to, either.) By the way, the average charge for a hospital-based vaginal delivery is $6,430 versus $11,000 for a c-section. Both figures include physician fees.

◆ *Do not routinely circumcise your male babies.*

Circumcision is an operative procedure for which hospitals charge between $124 to $148. It is recognized to be unnecessary for health reasons; consequently, more and more health insurance companies are refusing to pay for this procedure. For more information, contact

National Organization of Circumcision Information
    Resource Centers
P.O. Box 2512
San Anselmo, CA 94979-2512
415-488-9883
415-488-9660 (fax)

◆ *Demand itemized bills.*

Ongoing studies by national hospital bill auditing firms
consistently show that more than 90 percent of all hospital
bills contain errors—miscalculations that are seldom in your,
the consumer's, favor. In fact, the situation has gotten so out
of hand that businesses are now offering bounties to employees who can spot the inaccuracies in their bills. The reward is
a split of the money recovered from the hospital.

The problem here is that you can spot these errors only
if you receive an itemized bill, which in most cases, will not be
given to you unless you ask for it. Scrutinize the bill closely,
looking for any supplies, services, procedures or tests that
you did not receive.

If your bill is going to be paid by your insurer, be sure
to inform your insurer directly and in writing of any inaccuracies in the bill. Everyone saves money by making sure that
insurers do not overpay hospitals.

◆ *Keep a diary to compare with the hospital bill.*

Document all medications, tests and procedures and
compare your list with the itemized hospital bill. Make sure
that individual items match those you actually received and
that you are not billed for more items than you received.
Again, if you didn't use or undergo it, don't pay for it. You'll
find a complete hospital diary in the back of the book *Take
This Book to the Hospital With You* (Allentown, PA: People's
Medical Society, 1997), along with a hospital evaluation form
that should be sent to the People's Medical Society.

HOSPITAL BILLING ERRORS:
WHAT TO LOOK FOR

American Claims Evaluation, Inc., a firm in the business of auditing hospital bills, recommends that you ask yourself the following questions to help identify possible errors on a bill. Clearly, these do not cover every possible misbilling, but they are a good start.

1. Was I billed for the right kind of room (semiprivate, private, etc.)?

2. Was I billed for the correct number of days I occupied the hospital room?

3. Was I billed correctly for any time spent in specialized units (intensive care unit, coronary care unit, etc.)?

4. If I left before checkout time, was I billed for an extra day even though I'd already gone?

5. Was I billed only for those x-rays and tests that I actually received?

6. If I had preadmission testing, did the hospital bill me for the standard admission test battery even though I never had it?

7. Was I charged only for supplies, medications, therapy, dressings and injections that I received? Were the quantities correct?

8. Were medications that my doctor prescribed billed over the entire stay even though I took them only once or twice?

9. Were drugs prescribed for me to take home actually received?

10. Was I billed for bedpans, humidifiers, admission kits and thermometers that I never received and/or was not allowed to take home?

◆ *Ask for a daily bill.*

Hospital bills are long and confusing. If you are in a hospital for more than a day, ask to have a copy of the previous day's charges delivered to your room each morning. Like a fine hotel, hospitals keep a running tab of expenditures credited to your account. By asking to see a copy of the daily tab, you'll be better able to question certain charges that look wrong, suspicious or too high.

◆ *Make sure you get what you pay for.*

Many hospitals are teaching hospitals, which means they have a staff of medical interns and residents who work with "attending" physicians (such as your doctor). Unfortunately, this means that although you are paying full fees to your doctor, she may be doing very little of the work. You should specify, in writing, that any surgery or invasive procedure be done by the person you are paying for the service. If you are paying for a fully trained physician, that is who you should get.

◆ *Refuse to be seen by any doctor you don't know.*

If any doctor you do not know enters your hospital room to see you, you can be sure you will receive a bill for his services (often nothing more than a quick glance into your room) unless you immediately make it clear that you do not want those services. Find out who these doctors are and why they are there and make sure you or your insurer does not pay later for the services.

◆ *Have a friend or relative with you to act as advocate.*

In chapter 1, we suggested to always take a friend or relative with you into a doctor's examining room. It's just as important, maybe more important, to always have someone with you at the hospital. As a hospital patient, it is very difficult to be an assertive consumer. Always bring along a friend or family member to act as an advocate, whose most important task will be to make sure you do not agree to anything without fully understanding it. In many cases, these personal advocates may have to stay with you 24 hours a day.

Many hospitals have on staff a so-called patient advocate, who supposedly can help you resolve minor problems. While we can't vouch for the effectiveness of every patient advocate, it's a good idea to at least become acquainted with this person. Let this person know that you're an informed consumer and won't hesitate to call upon him if a situation should arise. And don't forget to bring to the hospital your copy of *Take This Book to the Hospital With You,* the People's Medical Society's guide to surviving your hospital stay.

◆ *Die at home.*

Over 50 percent of medical costs are incurred in the last five days of life. Of course, the decision about where to die is very personal and one that many never get the opportunity to make. But it is a valid consideration—for many reasons, including cost—and should be given serious thought.

◆ *Make a living will.*

A **living will** is a legal document that is used to inform family and medical personnel of your wishes concerning medical care, should you be unable to personally make those wishes known. These documents are most often used to limit the types of medical care you wish to receive if you are known to be in a terminal stage of illness. For instance, a living will may proscribe the use of an artificial life-sustaining treatment, such as an automatic ventilator. By law, every hospital is required to ask you if you have a living will or any other type of directive that can be followed if the issue should arise. The law does not require you to have such directives nor does it mean you must make one up. It merely requires hospitals to ask.

There are many reasons, in addition to the cost considerations, to choose to have a living will. No matter what your reasons, it is a good idea to discuss your living will with both your family and your doctor. And prepare your family to fight for your right to the choices expressed in the living will should you personally be unable to do so.

If you do have a living will, make sure you give a copy to your family doctor and any other physician you regularly use. If you are brought to a hospital unconscious or with no family member present, contact may be made with one of these doctors, who can then pass along your instructions.

To obtain more information on living wills and **durable power of attorney for health care**—another form of **advance directive**—contact:

> Choice in Dying
> 200 Varick St.
> New York, NY 10014
> 800-989-WILL

◆ *Bring your own food.*

Hospital meals are expensive (and, frankly, not always edible), partly because of the costs of hiring clinical dietitians who order menus based upon patients' nutritional needs. But if you are permitted to eat a normal diet, you will not need any special food and can save a lot of money—and keep your taste buds happy in the process—by providing your own food. (Skeptics of hospital food—and there are many, including probably most people who have ever eaten such food—maintain that you won't miss much.) This strategy may also be necessary if you are on a restricted diet, such as vegetarian or kosher. Remember, though, that providing three meals per day is hospital routine. So make it explicit that you do not want the meals and will not pay for them.

◆ Bring your own drugs.

As we noted earlier, this is a savvy (and easy) money-saving technique. Bring to the hospital an adequate supply of any medications you take (making sure beforehand, of course, that your doctor is aware of your usual medication regimen and has documented such in your hospital record). Medicate yourself at the appropriate times. It is also a good idea to take along some basic analgesics, such as aspirin or aceta-minophen, if you use them. Hospitals charge a lot ($3 for two aspirin tablets, in some cases) for medications.

If you are unable to medicate yourself, ask a family member to help. Have your doctor inform the nurses of such an arrangement.

◆ Bring your own vitamins to the hospital.

Hospitals do not ordinarily supply vitamin or mineral supplements—and if they did, you can be sure it would be at an exorbitant price. So if you customarily follow a vitamin and mineral supplementation regimen, bring your vitamins with you. And make sure the doctor marks on your chart that you are to be given your own vitamins or that supplements are to stay in your possession so you can take them yourself.

◆ Avoid weekend admission.

Don't allow yourself to be admitted on a nonemergency basis on a Friday afternoon or evening. You will just languish, expensively and in no particular comfort, until Monday. Most of the labs that would be performing your diagnostic workups don't do those things on weekends. Weekend admission equals one or two days extra in the hospital, at your expense. Only basic care is performed on the weekend. Wait until Monday—better yet, Tuesday, some experts say. By Tuesday, the hospital is back in gear after the weekend and the end-of-the-week blahs haven't hit yet.

◆ *Complain if you are being disturbed.*

Hospital personnel are accustomed to dealing with un-complaining, often drugged, patients. If your room is noisy at night or your sleep is disturbed, complain. A *British Medical Journal* report some years back cited more than 20 studies that responded resoundingly yes to the question "Is sound, prolonged sleep essential for optimal healing?" The savvy medical consumer will make sure that adequate rest periods of uninterrupted sleep are part of the care plan.

◆ *When in doubt, seek out the best hospital for your condition.*

All hospitals are not alike. As we noted earlier in this chapter, finding a hospital that frequently performs the procedure you need is a good way to improve your chances of a successful outcome. But what if there is no hospital (or doctor, for that matter) in your area that has an extensive amount of experience doing the operation or procedure you need? What do you do?

The savvy medical consumer will look nationally for what the medical world calls the centers of excellence for a particular procedure. For example, you probably know that Memorial Sloan Kettering Hospital in New York City is known for cancer treatment. Or that the Mayo Clinic in Rochester, Minnesota, has a worldwide reputation for diagnostics. Just because you do not live where one of these highly regarded institutions is located does not mean you cannot or should not have access to them. In fact, if no one locally is sure of your problem or if no one has a great deal of experience treating it, it's time to look elsewhere.

There are a number of publications, including a book published by *U.S. News and World Report,* that rank the best hospitals in America. While this is highly subjective, it does give you an idea of places to turn to for help. Also, don't be afraid to ask your doctor about a center of excellence outside your local area. You might also contact a medical school in your state, or one of national prominence, and ask for their recommendations of hospitals around the country that specialize in your problem.

◆ Use a community hospital for your routine procedures.

Most of us think we need to go to the most renowned hospital for even routine procedures. But the fact is, studies show that community hospitals are usually just as good as, and maybe better than (we'll tell you why in a moment), high-flying, heavily funded teaching hospitals. The reason is simple. Most hospitals today are high-tech institutions. Most can handle just about anything of a common nature that passes their portals. While teaching hospitals are excellent choices if you have a rare or complicated problem, they also tend to have higher infection rates, more medication errors and less personal service. You're more likely to be seen by a student, rather than a doctor, and the sheer volume of business that goes on in these medical behemoths tends to make you feel like a condition rather than a person. Plus, you are bound to pay a lot less in the community hospital.

So don't rush for the biggest and gaudiest when the smaller and simpler may be just your cup of tea.

Laboratories

Overtesting, unnecessary testing and errors in test results are problems you need to be on the lookout for. They can do irreparable harm to your pocketbook—*and your health,* if you undergo a dangerous invasive procedure as a result of a faulty test result. A former editor of one of the American Medical Association's journals has estimated that more than half of the tens of millions of medical tests performed annually "do not really contribute to a patient's diagnosis or therapy." And the Centers for Disease Control and Prevention has found that as many as 50 percent of simple blood and urine chemistry tests done in the top 10 percent of the laboratories in the United States are inaccurate. Lab tests can be expected to produce incorrect results a certain percentage of the time, so even the healthiest person will have an abnormal test result from time to time.

There's also the issue of defensive medicine. If the term is new to you, it is doctor-speak meaning, "I gotta do the test because if I don't, the litigious patient might later sue me if something goes wrong." Physicians are subjecting unsuspecting (and usually litigiously low-risk) customers to a battery of worthless pokes and probes that would send Hippocrates, if he were alive today, back to his famed oath ("First, do no harm") to add a new canon that would state, "Second, do no unnecessary test."

What can you do? Ensure that you have tests only when necessary and retest when appropriate. Here's how you do it.

◆ Avoid hospital laboratories and laboratories and imaging centers owned by doctors.

Hospital labs are no more reliable than independent laboratories, and they are usually considerably more expensive because the hospital overhead (cost of building, equipment and utilities) is higher.

Also, don't use a laboratory or imaging center that is owned by the physician making the referral. It just stands to reason. No judge should preside over a case in which she has a personal, vested interest. Ethics panels and the public just wouldn't stand for it. No government official should give contracts to friends, or hire relatives or purchase supplies from a company the official owns or has stock in. So why, then, let physicians refer patients to x-ray labs, specialty clinics, private hospitals, kidney dialysis units and physical therapy practices that these same physicians either own or have a financial interest in? Why permit this conflict of interest, ripe for exploitation of the consumer?

In medicine, it's called referral for profit, although more hard-nosed critics have labeled it a kickback scheme. Something else the savvy medical consumer *really* must be aware of: The latest evidence is that doctors who have a financial interest in laboratories order four times the number of diagnostic tests as physicians with no financial investment. And a General Accounting Office study found that physician-owners of Maryland labs or imaging centers ordered, on the average, 14 percent more expensive lab tests and 82 percent more expensive imaging tests than nonowner doctors.

How prevalent are these joint ventures, these investments in health-care facilities by physicians in positions to refer patients for tests or services? An important Florida study, released in August 1991, found that at least 40 percent of the doctors practicing in that state had invested in joint ventures to which they could refer patients. Regulations since then have reduced the overall number, but the consumer should still be on guard against the doctor who is more interested in protecting his investment than in healing the sick.

◆ Don't let the laboratory run more tests than you need.

You will notice that lab forms, particularly for blood and urine tests, list a number of different tests on one slip. Make sure that you and your doctor clearly indicate the specific tests that you need. Otherwise, the lab may run all the tests on the lab slip, and you will be charged for them.

Routine presurgical lab tests are another problem area. They account for at least $30 billion a year in business, yet researchers have found that nearly half the time, the tests duplicate those that patients had within the previous year. The findings indicate that normal results taken up to four months prior to surgery can be substituted safely for pre-operative screening tests.

◆ If your doctor recommends an invasive procedure as the result of a laboratory test, request a retest before agreeing to the procedure.

Because of the large number of errors made in laboratory tests, it makes sense both financially and for the sake of your health to pay the small fee for another lab test. Erroneous lab results can expose you to expensive, dangerous and potentially life-threatening invasive procedures. If your insurance plan requires approval for any retesting, just remind the powers-that-be that a $25 or even a $200 retest can save thousands in future expenses, not to mention out-of-pocket costs that are your responsibility.

◆ *Investigate the use of home tests rather than laboratory tests.*

Consumers are doing more to keep the doctor away, or at bay, than just eating an apple a day. Sales of do-it-yourself medical tests a few years ago topped the $500-million-a-year mark and climbed to $2.5 billion in 1996. Sold in drugstores, in supermarkets and through catalogs, home tests make it possible for you to take your own blood pressure, check yourself for a urinary tract infection, determine whether you're pregnant, screen yourself for certain cancers, detect the presence of the HIV virus, monitor your blood sugar levels and even predict when you're ovulating. In the early stages of diagnosis, home testing offers a low-cost, convenient alternative to the doctor's office or lab, with results that are quick and private.

But aside from the cost-containment angle, such testing is a good idea because it enables the consumer to involve herself in self-care and in aspects of health care once exclusively the doctor's domain. Do-it-yourself tests, however, are not without potential problems—accuracy, for one, and the situation in which your doctor just repeats the test you took at home. Most experts agree that the objective of home medical tests is for you to *work together* with your health professional to ensure the best health for yourself. Your pharmacist is a good source of information on home medical tests and can tell you what is presently available.

Remember, too, that not all home testing requires a kit. According to the American Cancer Society, every woman over 20 should examine her breasts monthly. Also, the most common type of cancer in humans, skin cancer, is largely curable if caught early, and you don't need a kit to check your skin for moles and suspicious and rapid changes in them.

◆ *Take advantage of free testing programs at community health fairs.*

Usually sponsored by hospitals and featuring lots of give-aways like refrigerator magnets and such, health fairs offer simple screening tests: blood pressure, cholesterol and tuberculosis screening; blood typing; screening for foot deformities and problems; vision testing; and on and on. Since these screenings are usually free, the greatest cost advantage to this method of testing is that you avoid having to pay for a doctor's visit unless one of the test results indicates that you need a doctor's care.

You should know that most health fairs are set up for the purpose of getting the consumer to use (translation: *buy*) the services of the participating providers, be they health-care facilities or physicians. In the words of a top medical marketer, writing in *Medical Economics*, "Doctors looking for an inexpensive way to attract more patients frequently sign up with health fairs...just the kind of low-key marketing that many physicians like best." In other words, keep a cautious attitude and make sure the fair promoters are providing a community service—not just an opportunity for doctors and hospitals to make a quick buck (or several hundred and more) off you.

◆ *Make sure the laboratory is certified.*

As we've noted, not all laboratories are equal in quality. One way to help ensure that your test or specimen is handled and analyzed correctly is to have the test performed at a laboratory certified by one of the agencies listed on page 19.

◆ *Find out when to expect results.*

Whenever a lab test is ordered, ask your doctor when to expect the results. When that day arrives, call the doctor first thing in the morning to remind him you expect a call that day with the outcome. Studies show that many doctors are not good about notifying patients, in a timely fashion, of their test results. In fact, many doctors have lost malpractice cases for not looking at the returned tests (and merely filing them in the patient's record) or not making an adequate effort to contact the patient with the findings. If you haven't heard from the doctor by 4 P.M. on the day results are expected, call again.

Insurance

Everyone hopes to stay healthy—but since there's a good chance that you or a member of your family will get sick at some point, it's smart to know how to shop for the best health insurance for your money.

Most people carry health insurance, if they can afford it, or have it provided as a benefit of employment. Lately, though, you've probably noticed that your coverage is not as extensive as it once was and you're paying more out-of-pocket expenses for deductibles and copayments. Some employers who once provided cost-free health insurance now require employees to make premium contributions.

While health insurance premiums have remained steady for the last few years (and in some cases, have even gone down slightly), the cost of health care is still rising and will continue to do so. That means that health insurance rates, whether for an indemnity plan or a managed-care plan, will ultimately go up. In addition, many companies, as a way to control their health-care expenditures for employees, have purchased health insurance plans that pay fewer benefits. This leaves you, the employee, facing larger and larger out-of-pocket expenses. The goal, then, is to maximize your health insurance benefits and reduce your out-of-pocket expenses as much as possible. Here's how.

◆ *Don't duplicate coverage.*

Chances are you will not be permitted to collect full benefits from both policies. The insurance companies invoke a policy they call **coordination of benefits**, which means they compare notes to determine who owes what. They split the bill, or at least the portion that is their responsibility, and you still must pick up any copayment or deductible. In essence, then, the premium for the second policy is down the drain.

◆ *Don't buy disease-specific or accident insurance.*

Disease-specific insurance usually covers one disease— for example, cancer or heart disease—and not only pays limited benefits, but may also duplicate what you already have or are about to purchase. Very limited in coverage (and for this reason, not the best insurance for your money), accident insurance excludes illness but does cover medical expenses resulting from an accident. And most insurers will not allow you to collect from more than one policy for a single injury.

◆ *Shop carefully for long-term-care insurance.*

This insurance is also known as nursing home insurance. The most important point to ask is whether benefits are paid for any level of care: skilled, intermediate or custodial (which usually includes assisted-living arrangements). It's important to make sure the policy you buy pays for all three levels. Up until a few years ago, long-term-care insurance paid benefits *only* for care in a **skilled nursing facility**, but today, policies usually cover the full range of services available. The benefits are paid when such services are deemed medically necessary.

◆ *Buy long-term-care insurance only if you have significant assets to protect.*

Many consumers are buying long-term-care insurance when they do not need it. You should buy a policy only if you have significant financial assets to protect, usually more than $100,000 plus your home. The reason *not to buy* with less than that is that the federal government, through the Medicaid program, pays for nursing home care, regardless of your age, if your assets are below a certain level. And with nursing home care costing anywhere from $30,000 to $80,000 per year, it does not take long for you to "spend down" to Medicaid levels. Thus, unless you have a lot of money to protect, it may be cheaper to pay for a year or so of nursing home care from your own assets and then go on Medicaid than to pay many years of fairly expensive premiums for long-term-care insurance.

So before you buy long-term-care insurance, talk it over with a financial planner or lawyer.

◆ *Take advantage of the free-look period.*

After you have signed an insurance application and paid the premium, your state may permit you to review the policy for a certain number of days—most allow 10 to 15 days—before you decide whether to keep it. If you are not satisfied and decide not to keep the policy, return it to the company within the time allotted and request a full refund of any premium. Call your state insurance department if you have any questions about your policy or about your state's free-look regulation.

◆ *Ask if your employer pays a bounty for erroneous medical bills.*

The first question a savvy medical consumer asks is, "How good are my chances of finding errors?" Companies that audit hospital bills for insurance companies report that over 90 percent of these bills have errors in them: the majority in favor of the hospital! When the *Philadelphia Daily News* took a look at billing—again, hospital bills, in particular—in that city, it found case after case of erroneous charges. In one case, a man had his $25,185 bill for a two-week hospital stay reduced by more than $2,000 after an auditor discovered overcharges.

Many companies will pay a reward, or bounty, to an employee who finds inaccuracies in her hospital bill that result in savings to the company. And as you can imagine, it shouldn't be too difficult to find an error. Your vigilance not only helps reduce your copayment, but your employer also benefits from the overall reduction in health insurance costs.

Don't be surprised if your insurer is not overly enthusiastic when you call to report a hospital's or doctor's overcharge. Insurance companies often find it easier to pay erroneous claims than to go to the trouble of auditing the bill and possibly demanding a refund. But you and everyone else pay for overcharges, so be persistent. Be prepared to fight with your insurer over an error in your bill.

◆ Get preapproval to make sure services are covered.

Nowadays, most insurance companies require preapproval for any major or costly procedure your doctor recommends. This applies to both managed-care plans as well as traditional fee-for-service and indemnity-type health insurance plans, which pay a set fee for a particular service. This just means that you (or your doctor) submit a request to your insurance company, who will then either approve or disapprove coverage for the recommended procedure. The process of preapproval becomes even more important when there are penalties attached to bypassing the system. You may opt to have a procedure or treatment done without approval only to learn that your coverage has been reduced by half (or in some cases, totally). Remember that no matter how insistent your doctor is, always check with your insurance carrier prior to any service to make sure the recommended procedure will be covered.

◆ *Pay premiums annually if you can afford to.*

You may be able to receive a discount on your premium if you can pay yearly in one lump sum or even on a semi-annual basis. If you don't have an insurance plan where you work, consider asking your employer to pick up part of your premium. This way, you can make the yearly premium payment and obtain a small benefit from your employment. It also saves your employer the full cost of starting a medical benefits plan.

◆ *Check out HMOs and PPOs—they may be cheaper than health insurance and may offer better benefits.*

HMOs and PPOs are forms of health insurance policies as well as providers. Managed-care plans (see chapter 6 for complete tips on managed care), as they are often called, are sometimes referred to as alternative delivery systems, which simply means alternatives to the traditional fee-for-service system. For the savvy medical consumer, the time to learn the rudiments of managed-care plans is *now*—as the popularity of these plans increases every year and more employers drop traditional insurance entirely and offer managed-care plans or nothing.

Health maintenance organizations come in a variety of forms, but with some elements in common:

▶ HMO members (usually called subscribers) receive comprehensive medical care for a fixed (or prepaid, meaning paid before you receive the services) monthly premium.

▶ The services are provided by an organized group of medical professionals who receive a fixed monthly payment per subscriber, regardless of the services rendered (or not rendered, whatever the case may be).

▶ Subscribers, for the most part, are limited to those physicians, hospitals and other medical providers approved by the HMO.

A preferred-provider organization is a group of physicians and hospitals that contract with insurance companies, unions or employers to provide health care at negotiated fees. In return, the preferred group is guaranteed a volume of patients.

You need to find out when the HMOs in your area have **open enrollment periods** and whether you meet the enrollment criteria. Also, speak to your employer about offering an HMO as an option to traditional health insurance—if your company does not already. If your company offers a PPO, be aware that by joining it, you may be severely limited in the providers you may use.

Consider what it would mean to you to change doctors or use a hospital that is not your favorite, should these be limitations set by the HMO or PPO. In either case, compare rates and coverage. HMOs and PPOs may (or may not) be cheaper.

◆ Use only providers who accept your insurance plan.

Some health insurers have arrangements with certain doctors and hospitals—called **participating providers**. Your policy will reimburse at a higher level if you use a participating provider.

◆ See if you're eligible for group insurance through organizations or associations to which you belong.

If you are unemployed or otherwise without an employer-subsidized health insurance policy, you may be able to obtain a less expensive group policy through organizations or associations to which you belong—and you may not have to look any farther than your mailbox. Many fraternal, alumni and civic associations have health insurance plans for sale. While many of these offerings are indemnity plans—i.e., they pay a fixed amount per day in the hospital or per service—in a pinch, they can cover at least some of your expenses.

Some states are now offering low-cost insurance for disabled and/or handicapped persons who are unable to obtain private insurance. Contact your state insurance department or department of welfare to see if it is available where you live and if you are eligible.

◆ Donate blood—join a blood bank.

By committing yourself to the donation of a specified amount of blood per year, you can receive insurance coverage for blood supplies for yourself and possibly for your family as well.

◆ Join an ambulance service.

Just as with a blood bank, private and voluntary ambulance services often offer a specified amount of service for a yearly donation.

◆ Check all employer-sponsored health insurance plan options carefully.

A happy scenario is one where your employer, as many larger companies are doing, offers a wide range of policies and options at varying costs. Many workers are offered a cafeteria package of benefits and must choose from an assortment of possibilities. Unfortunately, too many people decide by the toss of a coin—an uninformed and hardly savvy decision-making tactic. To get the best value for your money, carefully compare all the policies with *your needs* in mind. Do not settle for less coverage than you need. Your premium for more coverage may not be much higher.

◆ Pay premiums on time.

An insurance company can cancel your policy if you fail to pay the premium or continually pay the premium late. Be sure to keep on top of any necessary employee deductions if yours is an employer-sponsored policy.

◆ *Know what your state insurance department can do for you in the way of consumer protection.*

Your state insurance department plays an important role in regulating insurance companies. Beyond licensing insurance companies and agents, approving policies that are sold and mandating minimum benefits for policies, the department has the power to conduct investigations, take testimony, hold hearings and render verdicts. As such, your state insurance department may also be able to help you if you have a problem with an insurance company or agent. Any formal complaint you file with the department will be investigated and, if possible, resolved.

HOW TO FILE A COMPLAINT WITH YOUR STATE INSURANCE DEPARTMENT

Your complaint should be in writing and contain the following information:

▶ Your name, address and telephone number

▶ The name, address and telephone number of your insurance company

▶ The identification number of your policy

▶ The type of policy

▶ The nature of your complaint: the premium, the coverage, a claim or the actions of your agent

Make sure you keep copies of everything you send to the department. You must be willing to follow through on your complaint and appear at any hearings if so directed. If the law and the facts are on your side, the insurance department can usually help resolve the problem.

Managed Care

The biggest change in health care in the 1990s is the growth of managed care. From health maintenance organizations to **point-of-service (POS) plans,** managed care has become the dominant form of health insurance in America. At the end of 1996, more than 65 percent of all Americans were enrolled in some form of managed-care program. And even if you continue to be in a traditional indemnity health insurance plan, the chances are it has managed-care elements.

Managed care is not a new concept. Its roots go back more than 50 years, when some large employers wanted to provide high-quality health-care services to their employees but wanted to control the cost and quality of the services. It didn't take off in a big way until medical inflation hit double digits in the 1980s and employers and the federal government were seeing staggering annual increases in their medical costs.

All managed care is not the same. In fact, the quality varies from plan to plan and even within some plans. The savvy medical consumer is the person who knows what to look for when choosing a managed-care plan and how to make the plan work for her once enrolled. Polls show that generally those enrolled in managed-care programs like their plans. The numbers drop some, though, if the consumer is confronted with a serious illness. That is when the real test of a plan's quality and service is seen. But if you do your homework in advance, the chances are that managed care can be a very helpful and healthful way to get your health care.

◆ Consider managed-care programs.

Managed care is a form of health insurance. No matter what the managed-care model (see below), the goals of managed care are the same. Managed care is designed to provide only the health care you need, at a price you can afford. Physicians are paid either a salary or a monthly fee no matter how many visits or services you receive. Therefore, the incentive to make more money by providing unnecessary services is removed. At the same time, managed care tends to be more prevention-oriented than the traditional fee-for-service or indemnity insurance models. Simply, managed-care companies make more money if you stay well. Consumers in most managed-care programs give their plans high ratings. Features they particularly like are the level of coverage, the security of knowing what their medical costs will be for the full year and the prevention orientation of the programs.

◆ Understand the various types of managed care.

In addition to HMOs, PPOs and POSs, there are also **physician hospital organizations (PHOs)** and **Medicare and Medicaid HMOs**.

HMOs are the oldest and easiest type of managed care to understand. Consumers using an HMO program become members of a particular HMO plan. There are now hundreds of them all across the country. As a member, you or your employer pays the HMO company a monthly premium. For that premium, you receive all the medical care you need. That includes both physician and hospital services. It often includes services not usually covered, or fully covered, by fee-for-service or indemnity insurance plans, such as immunizations, mammograms and well-baby visits. In return for receiving these services, the member agrees to use only those doctors or medical facilities affiliated with or employed by the HMO. If, at any time, you use a doctor or hospital not affiliated with the HMO, you will be responsible for the entire cost of that service yourself.

HMOs can be either nonprofit entities or for-profit companies. They come in two forms, **staff model** and **open panel**. Under the staff model, the HMO actually employs its own physicians, paying each an annual salary and possibly a bonus. In the open panel HMOs, private physicians are contracted by the HMO to provide services to its members. Under this model, each physician receives a monthly reimbursement for every HMO member who selects his practice, whether services are rendered or not. Most HMOs are open panel models.

PPOs are the same as HMOs except that they are owned by the physicians in the program. While they tend to offer the same services as an HMO, PPOs may not have as many doctors or hospitals to choose from. They may also have a limited number of services available outside your local area (a consideration if you travel or have children at school away from home).

POS plans are a cross between an HMO and the fee-for-service or indemnity health insurance plan. In fact, a POS plan is the best of both worlds. In this model, you or your employer pays a monthly premium to a managed-care company. If you use the company's doctors and hospitals, you pay nothing more (other than a possible small copayment per doctor visit). However, if you go outside its network of doctors and hospitals, the insurer will still pay a significant portion of the bill, usually 60 to 70 percent. You must pay the difference. On the other hand, your out-of-pocket costs are capped. Usually, the cap is between $1,000 and $2,500 per year. After you have paid that amount in a given year, the insurer picks up the rest.

PHOs are a recent addition to managed care. Few in number, they are like a PPO except that they are owned by hospitals and the doctors affiliated with them. The advantages are that members tend to receive services at the same facilities and often are provided services not otherwise provided by a PPO or an HMO that covers multiple facilities. The disadvantage is that these arrangements are often very local and narrow in the number of doctors and hospitals participating.

Medicare and Medicaid HMOs are exactly what their names imply: HMOs approved by the federal Health Care Financing Administration for Medicare and Medicaid beneficiaries' participation.

◆ *Review managed-care programs carefully.*

Be careful when selecting a managed-care program. Check out the company that owns the program. Has it been in the managed-care business a long time? Are the rules of the program clear and easily understood? Are you satisfied with the list of doctors and hospitals available? Be sure you know exactly what is covered and what is not. This is particularly important if you or a family member has a chronic condition or is anticipating a particular type of care in the future. Remember that no two managed-care companies or programs are alike.

◆ *Don't join a newly formed managed-care program.*

Wait until the program has been up and running in *your community* for at least four years. Even if the program is part of a large national organization such as Kaiser or Oxford, give the local program time to get established. When a managed-care program is started locally, the owners must recruit doctors and hospitals. Often, they take what they can get or what other managed-care companies have passed over.

So, let the company "mature" in your area before you sign on the dotted line.

◆ *Know the program's policy on emergency care.*

Ideally, the managed-care company will want you to use its emergency center (if it has one) or an affiliated hospital's emergency room. But emergencies don't always happen at locations convenient to these sites. Today, most HMOs and other managed-care programs tell you to go directly to an emergency room. Usually, on the back of your membership card is a toll-free phone number for you or emergency personnel to call once you or your family member is stabilized. But be sure to get, in writing, what you must do to make sure an emergency visit is covered under the program.

◆ *Know your rights when out of town.*

Even though many managed-care companies are owned by major corporations and are national in scope, most programs have different rules in each locality. One reason for this is that managed care, in any form, is regulated by state insurance departments. Since each state has differing laws governing managed-care programs, a Prudential program in Pennsylvania, for example, may have different rules than a Prudential program in Illinois. This becomes important if you travel on business or vacation out of the local area. Be sure you understand what you have to do if you need medical attention while away from home. Ask for it in writing and take a copy with you when you are on your trip. Also, be careful when you travel overseas. In most cases, your insurance or managed-care contract will not pay for care you receive outside the United States. You may need to buy travelers' health insurance before you depart.

◆ *Check out doctors and hospitals.*

When you enter a managed-care program, you basically agree to use its doctors and facilities for a set monthly premium. If you go outside its network of providers, you will either pay a significant portion of the cost or all of it. Therefore, it is essential that you are comfortable with the doctors and facilities in the program.

Check out the following before you make the decision to join:

DOCTORS

▶ Make sure all primary-care doctors and specialists are board certified in their specialties. (See page 15.)

▶ Don't join a managed-care program that has fewer than three doctors in any specialty or fewer than 10 primary-care physicians.

▶ Be sure you can pick any doctor on the list. Sometimes, physicians limit the number of patients they take from any given managed-care program. Check to see if the practice you're interested in using is open to new patients.

▶ Find out what happens when your doctor is unable to see you or is on vacation. Who is the backup practitioner?

HOSPITALS

▶ Be sure all the hospitals in the program are accredited by the Joint Commission on the Accreditation of Healthcare Organizations. (See page 92.)

▶ Check to be sure that at least one of the hospitals has an extensive department in the specialty areas you may use.

▶ Find out if the managed-care company contracts with hospitals with national reputations for certain specialties outside your local area. This is extremely important if you need high-level or cutting-edge technology for less common or more severe conditions.

◆ Know how to appeal decisions.

One major complaint about managed-care programs is that doctors and patients often don't have the final decision about treatments. Unlike the traditional fee-for-service insurance plans in which doctors and their patients jointly decide what the course of treatment will be, managed-care plans must approve those decisions. Doing so is the heart of managed care. By reviewing decisions doctors make, managed-care companies are monitoring to be sure they are the best and most appropriate courses of treatment. In most cases, the managed-care companies agree totally with a doctor's decision or recommendation. But there are instances when they do not. In those cases, the managed-care companies deny that service to the patient. However, that is not the end of it.

By law, every licensed managed-care company must have an appeals procedure that patients can use to overturn a negative decision or have it reviewed. The procedure varies from company to company and state to state. So, it is essential that you know and understand how to file such an appeal and what your rights are in the process. Anecdotal reporting suggests that consumers win a large percentage of these appeals.

◆ *Learn how to file a grievance.*

At times, you may be dissatisfied with the way a managed-care company is doing business. For example, you may have been told a certain type of procedure is covered, only to be told later it is not. There are two ways to handle grievances of this nature. One is to find out if your managed-care company has a formal grievance procedure. If it does, use it.

The second option is to file a formal complaint with your state's insurance department. The state insurance department, usually located in your state's capital, licenses every managed-care company. Your insurance department has formal procedures for dealing with complaints and grievances against managed-care entities. Find out your rights under these provisions in your state.

◆ *Watch out for medical malpractice.*

Managed care is merely an insurance program, so it is important to recognize that doctors and hospitals are still individual entities and do make mistakes. While many managed-care companies take great care in selecting doctors and choosing hospitals, they cannot stand over them as care is given. Therefore, it is important that you stay alert to errors or negligence that might be occurring in your treatment. Don't hesitate to inform the managed-care company if you suspect a practitioner or facility is not performing at the highest levels. Also, feel free to file a complaint with the medical or hospital licensing board in your state.

Watch what you sign concerning medical malpractice when you enroll in a managed-care company. Some companies make you agree not to sue the managed-care company if a physician or facility commits malpractice against you. They usually make you agree to an arbitration process. The record to date shows that in some of these arrangements, consumers actually win more malpractice cases than they do in court, but they usually win less money. So before you enroll, be careful to know exactly what your rights to redress are if you suspect medical malpractice has occurred in your course of care.

◆ *Look for an accredited managed-care program.*

With the growth of managed-care programs in the past decade, concern has grown about quality care. In recent years, a number of organizations have entered the business of accrediting managed-care programs. Check to see if the program you are considering is accredited by any of the following organizations:

> Accreditation Association for Ambulatory Healthcare
> 9933 Lawler, Suite 512
> Skokie, IL 60077-3702
> 708-676-9610

> Joint Commission on the Accreditation of
>   Healthcare Organizations
> One Renaissance Blvd.
> Oakbrook Terrace, IL 60181
> 630-916-5600

National Committee for Quality Assurance
2000 L St., N.W., Suite 500
Washington, DC 20036
202-955-3500

◆ *Look for features that help ensure quality care.*

Make sure the managed-care company has programs
that help to ensure quality care. For example, you should be
allowed to seek a second opinion on any diagnosis or recommended treatment. This is especially important if surgery or
some other **invasive treatment** regimen is suggested. There
should also be a provision for you to go outside the company's network of physicians when special expertise is needed
and is unavailable within the network. This latter point is
tricky, since most managed-care programs try to sell themselves as having everything you need. Usually, they do not, so
check out the company's policy about seeking independent
second opinions.

Also, find out how often the company reviews the overall
records of the hospitals and doctors with whom it contracts.
For example, does the managed-care company know each
hospital's infection or drug error rate? Does the company
know the rates of death and complications, by procedure,
of each of the doctors in its employ? Having this kind of information is vital to maintaining and improving quality of
care. Ask to see what the managed-care company does to
maintain quality.

◆ *Beware of slick-talking salespeople.*

Health care is first and foremost a business. In fact, it is
now the largest business in the United States. And managed
care is one of the most competitive parts of the health-care
business. Today, consumers can choose managed care from a
variety of insurance companies. The programs are made
available either directly to the consumer or through employers, service or fraternal organizations and unions. No matter

where you make the purchase, beware of managed-care-company sales agents. While most are honest, they are, in fact, just that—salespeople. In order to make the sale, managed-care sales agents have been known to exaggerate services, customer satisfaction levels and even levels of coverage. To be safe, *don't believe a word they say*, unless they can back it up in writing. Be especially leery of insurance brokers who contract, for a commission, with managed-care companies and serve as local agents. Many of these brokers represent more than one company, and while a broker may be able to find a managed-care program that's appropriate to your needs, he may also have an inherent conflict of interest because he would rather sell you the program that pays him the highest commission.

◆ Interview your prospective doctor before enrollment.

This is not something most managed-care companies encourage or even tolerate, but insist on doing it. Remember that the most important components of any managed-care program are its doctors and hospitals. Before enrolling, review the list of primary-care doctors in the network and tentatively note the practices you might select. Ask to set up an interview appointment with each practice. (See page 16.) If you know you will need a specialist because of an ongoing problem, do the same thing. It is not always easy to drop out of a managed-care program once you have signed a contract, and most employers limit the number of provider changes you can make.

◆ Look for additional services.

Many managed-care programs offer services above and beyond their basic coverage. Most have managed prescription drug programs you may purchase. Some provide managed vision care and dental coverage. Some or all of these additional covered services may be included. If not, ask about them. More often than not, these extra coverages are cheaper than what you would purchase outside the managed-care program and can offer substantial savings.

◆ *Make suggestions.*

This may sound strange, but don't hesitate to make recommendations to your managed-care company about service, coverage and practitioners. Remember that whether profit-making or not-for-profit, managed-care companies are big businesses. And businesses are always worried about losing customers, especially managed-care and health-care companies. If bad news is spread about one of these companies, it can go out of business in a flash. This is especially good news for medical consumers because it means that most managed-care companies are responsive to your suggestions. So make them. Tell them how their businesses could be run better. Let them know about staff with bad attitudes, bills that are unreadable, explanations that cannot be translated into any language. The more they hear, the more responsive they will be.

◆ *Don't hesitate to quit.*

If the managed-care program is not working for you, quit it. Of course, make sure you can leave without creating a gap in your medical insurance coverage. If you are employed and your employer allows switching only at a certain time of year, talk to the personnel or benefits director or the company owner. Maybe your problem is one shared by all of the company's employees. A call to the managed-care company from your boss might change it. Short of that, make your case as to why you need to switch before the end of the program year or arrival of the switching period. Also, be careful about expecting to reenroll in a fee-for-service insurance program if you have a preexisting condition. The new insurer may deny or limit your coverage. Check it out before you leave the managed-care program.

◆ *Organize a subscriber group.*

As already noted, most managed-care companies are very sensitive to member complaints or grievances. One way to maximize your power is to create a subscriber group, made up of your coworkers or others who belong to the same managed-care program. Group power is always greater than that of an individual, and it definitely will catch the attention of the managed-care company. Start small and meet once a month. Use your company newsletter to advertise the group's creation. Let the managed-care company know you have organized the group. Ask to have the managed-care company send representatives when you want specific answers to questions. Also, let the group be a way to help educate members. Have the managed-care company send someone to explain how it chooses member doctors or why certain hospitals are in (or out) of the program. Don't be afraid to confront the management with problems or suggestions that come forward in these sessions. Remember that it's your program, and it should be responsive to your needs and those of the other subscribers.

Long-Term Care, Nursing Homes and Home Health Care

Since the early 1990s, there has been a revolution in the nursing home industry. For starters, the terminology has changed. Today, most nursing homes are called long-term-care facilities. While most still provide some level of medical/nursing care, there are now many different models from which a consumer can choose. The models vary in the level of care provided. Some provide high-level medical care (skilled nursing facilities); others are little more than congregate living arrangements with minimal medical services available. And because of the aging of the American population, long-term-care facilities are the fastest-growing segment of the entire health-care system.

The term "nursing home" is actually a very general name for several different types of medical/long-term-care facilities. It has the connotation of being a last stop for the elderly, but it can actually be a place for people of all ages to convalesce following an accident or serious illness or a temporary placement for an older person while the family shops around and lines up alternative long-term modes of care. A common classification for nursing homes is the level of care they provide:

▶ *Skilled nursing.* Care is delivered by registered and licensed practical nurses on the orders of an attending physician. The person who requires a **skilled nursing facility** is often bedridden and not able to help himself.

▶ *Intermediate care.* The **intermediate-care facility** provides less intensive care than the skilled facility and usually costs less; the care there stresses rehabilitation therapy to enable the resident to go home or at least regain or retain as many functions of daily living as possible. Care is delivered by registered and licensed practical nurses and an array of therapists.

▶ *Assisted living, sheltered or **custodial care**.* This level of care is nonmedical in that residents do not require constant attention from nurses or aides but do need help with such routine activities as getting out of bed, walking, eating and bathing.

At some point over a lifetime, one in every five people can expect to need extended nursing care. To make matters worse, very few *basic* health insurance policies cover nursing home care for more than a few days or weeks. Even Medicare, the federal health insurance plan for senior citizens, does not cover what we think of as long-term care. Medicare covers a limited number of days of skilled nursing facility care only and is primarily intended to permit recovery outside of a hospital. So if you or a member of your family needs such care, you must know how to get quality long-term care without paying more than necessary.

What follow are ways for the savvy medical consumer to get the best value in extended nursing care. Knowing all of your options is the key.

◆ *Use home health care.*

Home health agencies can provide services ranging from help with cooking and cleaning to full nursing care at home. For the elderly person with minor disabilities, a person to cook or clean is often all the support that's needed. A home health agency can help you evaluate the help that you need. But don't purchase any more care than necessary.

Bear in mind that home health care is not just for the elderly on Medicare. Many people under age 65, who are not yet legally disabled—and who, therefore, would not normally qualify for Medicare—but who require rehabilitative or chronic care, are eligible to use home care programs. Home health services offer an opportunity for early discharge from a hospital or a skilled nursing facility, and in fact, such specialized or rehabilitation services often meet a person's long-term needs more efficiently than acute care hospital settings.

If you are eligible for Medicare, know the limits of coverage of home health care. If you are not on Medicare, find out what your insurance plan pays and what eligibility requirements you must meet. Generally, a doctor must arrange for such services as part-time home nursing care, occupational therapy, speech therapy and special meals and other nutritional services to be furnished in your home.

◆ *Check the yellow pages for the visiting nurse association and other agencies that provide home health care.*

The first thing to know is that nursing home placement is not, and should not be, the sole solution to the plight of an older person who is debilitated by ill health and who has increasing difficulty taking care of herself. Nothing mandates nursing home placement if there is someone available to administer the needed care in the home or to coordinate delivery of alternative services. Visiting nurse associations (VNAs) are the oldest home health-care agencies in most communities; however, they aren't the only agencies that provide home health services. Hospitals, nonprofit community organizations and for-profit agencies are also in the home care business. VNAs provide referrals to other community services when appropriate.

Familiarize yourself with the various levels of care available in your community. Full-service agencies, such as the VNA and certified home health agencies, offer everything from skilled nursing care to homemaker services. If you're responsible for the full cost of the services, don't contract for more care than you need. Another important point to consider is whether the agency is certified. This could become rather important if your health insurance plan will cover services only from a certified agency. These groups can provide you with information on certified home care agencies:

Joint Commission on the Accreditation of
    Healthcare Organizations
One Renaissance Blvd.
Oakbrook Terrace, IL 60181
630-916-5600

National League for Nursing
350 Hudson St.
New York, NY 10014
212-989-9393

For information on home health services, contact:

Foundation for Hospice and Home Care
519 C St., N.E.
Washington, DC 20002
202-547-6586

◆ *Use adult day care.*

An adult day-care center lets an elderly person enjoy a full range of activities—including arts and crafts, games and just plain old conversation—on a daily basis in a supervised setting. Communities nationwide are establishing such facilities, which provide a degree of supervision and appropriate activities for elderly persons with minor physical disabilities but do not provide nursing care.

It is well established that elderly people remain healthier if they are able to continue to live in their own homes—and it's usually cheaper. Adult day care can often make the difference between being able to remain at home and needing institutionalization.

◆ *If you need nursing home care, purchase the lowest level necessary.*

Of the three levels of nursing home care—skilled, intermediate and assisted living—skilled care is the most expensive because the care is provided by registered and licensed practical nurses on the orders of an attending physician. Remember that skilled care is the only level of care that Medicare will reimburse for, and then only a very limited amount of coverage is provided.

For information on nursing home care, contact

> American Association of Homes and Services
>   for the Aging
> 901 E St., N.W., Suite 500
> Washington, DC 20004
> 202-783-2242

> American Health Care Association
> 1201 L St., N.W.
> Washington, DC 20005
> 202-842-4444

> National Consumers League
> 1701 K St., N.W., Suite 1200
> Washington, DC 20006
> 202-835-3323

QUICK CHECKLIST OF QUESTIONS FOR LONG-TERM-CARE/NURSING HOME ADMINISTRATORS

Even before you spend your time going around to various nursing homes and other long-term-care facilities, touring them and interviewing administrators, you should conduct phone interviews to establish a base of information on which to build. You will want to find out these things:

1. What level of care is offered?

2. Are there restrictions on the types of patients accepted?

3. How many beds (for the type of care you need) does the home provide?

4. Is there a waiting list, and if so, approximately how long is it?

5. What type of license or accreditation does the home have?

6. Does the home accept Medicare and Medicaid?

7. Is there an initial deposit required, and if so, how much is it?

8. What are the monthly room charges?

9. Are additional monthly services provided? What are their charges?

◆ *Use Meals on Wheels and/or other programs that are alternatives to institutionalization.*

An excellent program designed to provide hot, nutritious meals to homebound older people, Meals on Wheels is usually operated by a social service agency or community group. The service delivers one hot meal a day directly to the person's residence, and the price of such a service is nominal, often based on ability to pay.

As with a number of other programs for those people who do not require constant supervision or that much nursing care, Meals on Wheels may actually delay a person's need for a nursing home for many years. The savvy medical consumer will explore the other programs as well: *homemaker services,* for people who require some assistance in the preparation of meals or with housework; *home sharing,* an arrangement in which a resident manager and a few older people share housing and share expenses; *telephone reassurance,* a formal or informal system to take away the risk of total isolation for the elderly person living alone; *shopping services,* which entail having groceries and other needed items delivered; *special transportation services,* consisting of vehicles equipped to handle wheelchairs and other devices for people with limited mobility; and *special health aids or devices,* such as walkers, mechanical feeding devices, geriatric chairs and artificial limbs, which can facilitate personal independence or make it more feasible for a family member to assist. Contact your local, county or state welfare or human services agencies for availability of or more information about these programs.

◆ *Use a hospice.*

Hospices are for people who are terminally ill, and their mission is to promote death with dignity and allow the family close contact with the patient, free from the intrusive high technology of the hospital. Less expensive than a hospital because it does not use life-sustaining technologies, a hospice provides basic medical care, counseling for the patient and family and prescribed pain relievers. Most hospices will care for patients for whom a doctor's prognosis indicates fewer than six months to live. Some hospices come to a person's home and provide services, while others actually operate a facility where the patient resides. For information on hospice care, contact:

Children's Hospice International
2202 Mt. Vernon Ave., Suite 3-C
Alexandria, VA 22301
800-242-4453

Hospice Education Institute
Five Essex Sq., Suite 3-B
Essex, CT 06426-0713
800-331-1620

National Hospice Organization
1901 N. Moore St., Suite 901
Alexandria, VA 22209
800-658-8898

◆ *Investigate assisted living/life-care communities.*

A relatively new concept, these communities provide residential care in an apartment-like setting, along with skilled and intermediate nursing care. As residents require nursing care, they are transferred to the nursing home section of the community and, once they recover, return to their apartments. The life-care community covers all costs of hospitalization, so as you can imagine, the services do not come cheap. This option often requires a substantial, nonrefundable down payment as well as monthly fees. Two good sources of information on life-care communities are the following:

American Association of Homes and Services
for the Aging
901 E St., N.W., Suite 500
Washington, DC 20004
202-783-2242

Assisted Living Facilities Association of America
9411 Lee Hwy., Suite J
Fairfax, VA 22031
703-691-8100

◆ *Prepare for the financial costs of nursing care.*

Nursing home care is expensive, costing anywhere from $30,000 to $80,000 per year, depending on the level of care. Many insurance companies are now offering long-term-care insurance—specifically designed to cover nursing home care. If you're going to purchase such a policy, a good rule of thumb is to select a policy that pays at least $80 per day for nursing facility care and $40 a day for home care for four years of coverage. If you can afford it, add a 5 percent compounded inflation coverage rider to the policy. Look for a policy that will keep up with inflation. A present benefit of $60 a day could easily dwindle to a future value of only $20 due to inflation. To obtain a list of insurance companies offering long-term-care policies, contact

> Health Insurance Association of America
> 555 13th St., N.W., Suite 600-E
> Washington, DC 20004
> 202-824-1600

◆ *Find out if you're eligible for Medicaid.*

Medicaid, the government program for the poor, is the largest payer of long-term-care services in the country. The chances are that your friends and neighbors who have been in long-term-care programs for a while are having most of the bill paid by Medicaid! In 1995, Medicaid paid for more than $35 billion in nursing home and other institutional care and more than $12 billion in home and community-based services.

Medicaid is the government health insurance program that will pay for nursing home care when most of a person's assets have been depleted. The program generally pays for all levels of care in certified facilities for an indefinite period of time. It can include care in an assisted living or nursing facility.

Contact your state welfare department, area agency on aging or state department on elderly affairs to find out eligibility requirements in your state. Even if you are not eligible before you enter a nursing home, you will most likely become eligible if you "spend down" your assets in a long-term-care facility.

ARE YOU A CANDIDATE FOR LONG-TERM-CARE INSURANCE?

Not everyone is a candidate for long-term-care insurance. Currently, about half of those age 65 or older are unable to purchase coverage because of either their health or their inability to afford the premiums.

Money magazine suggests buying long-term-care insurance if you (and your spouse) are around age 65, your net worth is greater than $100,000 excluding your home and your annual income is at least $50,000 per year. We would also add that you should be in good health; otherwise, noncoverage for preexisting conditions could mean you never collect benefits.

Individuals with family histories of debilitating diseases such as stroke or Alzheimer's disease may want to consider coverage because the odds of needing nursing facility care are increased.

On the other hand, if you have the discipline to take the money that would be spent on the annual premiums ($1,000 to $3,000 per person per year starting at age 65) and invest it, the cash could give you greater flexibility than the insurance policy in later years in selecting long-term-care options.

◆ *Investigate any facility thoroughly before saying yes.*

Even if a long-term-care facility is licensed and certified, check it out carefully. Inspect it yourself. Look around. Are residents involved in constructive activities, or are they sitting around in wheelchairs staring off into space? Are they restrained in their beds or chairs more as a convenience to staff rather than out of danger of injury? Talk to other people who have family members in the facility. Find out their likes and dislikes about the staff, activities and medical care. Don't be shy about asking questions and sticking your nose into things. Remember that you can't be there every hour of every day looking after your loved one. Make sure you trust those running the place and working in it.

◆ *Make surprise visits to long-term-care facilities.*

The best way to know what goes on in a long-term-care facility is to visit it when you are not expected. Drop by late at night. See what's going on when residents are being awakened in the early morning. Come back an hour after you normally leave. Many nursing facilities operate well when they know an outside eye is on them, such as during normal visiting hours or when the state is coming to inspect. It's the rest of the time that you need to worry about. Don't be afraid to be a pain in the administration's side when it comes to assuring your loved one's care.

Medical Equipment

Durable medical equipment such as hospital beds and wheelchairs can be extremely valuable tools in caring for an ill person at home—*and* can save you money in the process. Anything that enables a sick person to remain at home rather than in an institution makes dollars and sense.

Now, the bad news. According to recent government reports, some unethical medical equipment companies have targeted Medicare beneficiaries as easy marks for purchasing medical equipment. The scam usually starts with a letter or telephone call to beneficiaries telling them that they are eligible for a particular piece of medical equipment and that Medicare will pay for it. The problem here is that the equipment may or may not be needed, and if it isn't medically necessary, Medicare will not pay for it. And guess who gets stuck with the bill?

If you know what to do, you can save money on durable medical equipment. Here are our suggestions.

◆ Borrow medical equipment whenever possible.

Most home health aids can be borrowed from various community organizations. Ask your local home health organization or visiting nurse association. If no such services are available in your area, you may be able to rent the required equipment from a local pharmacy. But before renting, check to see if your insurance policy will cover its purchase. Also, shop around; rental prices for equipment vary from dealer to dealer. If you need the equipment for a long period of time, you will probably have to purchase it.

◆ Save by owning medical self-care equipment.

Simple items of self-care equipment such as thermometers, blood pressure cuffs, stethoscopes and otoscopes are helpful devices, especially when it comes to making informed choices concerning your need for a doctor's help. Many are available from discount mail-order companies. Check out a number of suppliers to find a high-quality item at a reasonable price.

◆ Check out the equipment's reliability before purchasing.

Every piece of equipment should come with literature that describes its reliability within a certain range. For instance, thermometers may be reliable within a range of one degree Fahrenheit. Some equipment will be more reliable than others. The equipment's accompanying literature should also describe the period of time the equipment can be expected to maintain this degree of reliability without servicing.

Also, before purchasing a piece of durable medical equipment, find out about the warranty. Check, too, if the manufacturer or dealer offers extended warranty protection on particularly expensive items.

◆ Find out where servicing is available.

Equipment such as blood pressure cuffs must be periodically serviced to maintain reliability. Make sure that you know how, where and how often a piece of equipment must be serviced before you purchase it. In fact, it makes sense to purchase only equipment with a written warranty. Further, you will save money if the equipment you buy can be serviced locally.

◆ *Check out the supplier with the Better Business Bureau and with Medicare if the equipment is for a Medicare beneficiary.*

For many health items such as hearing aids, it is wise to see if your local Better Business Bureau has any complaints on file against the supplier from whom you are thinking of purchasing. If the equipment is prescribed for a Medicare beneficiary, determine if the supplier is a certified Medicare supplier. What this means is that the supplier will accept the Medicare-approved amount as payment in full and will bill the beneficiary only for the 20 percent copayment.

◆ *Check for sales.*

With health and medical equipment, just as with most other consumer items, suppliers often offer sales. Purchasing items on sale is always a good way to save money.

◆ *Return any medical equipment that arrives unsolicited.*

Some doctors and medical suppliers target Medicare beneficiaries with offers of so-called free equipment paid for by Medicare. In addition, some equipment manufacturers use well-known personalities to hawk various products ranging from special beds to power-assisted chairs. Be aware that Medicare will pay only for durable medical equipment that's prescribed by your doctor, as long as it is medically necessary. The words "medically necessary" are the key here. Unless your doctor specifically orders equipment, do not respond to any mail-order or telephone marketing schemes.

Prevention

Taking preventive measures has the potential to save you more money on health costs than anything else you do. Even more important, prevention is health promotion, something every savvy medical consumer should be doing more of. But the bad news is that while 58 cents out of every health-care dollar goes to doctors and hospitals, only two cents goes to health promotion activities. That's all we spend to keep ourselves healthy.

However, you have many opportunities in daily living to get your two cents' worth by doing things that will improve your health. And remember that the sooner you start, the healthier you will be.

◆ Learn stress-reduction techniques.

There are techniques—some simple, others requiring professional help—that can help you lower your stress level. Strong evidence exists that those under stress, or those who cope poorly with stress, are less healthy than others. And at the very least, that adds up to a lot of extra dollars spent on medical care.

◆ *Quit smoking.*

Smoking increases a person's risk for a number of major diseases: heart disease, stroke and cancer. But beyond that, smokers are just generally more prone to illness—and, therefore, lose more work time due to illness—than nonsmokers. If you are a smoker, consider also the increased risk at which you put your friends and family as they breathe in your exhaled smoke. Save money and your health by throwing away your cigarettes. And don't think that cigar or pipe smoking is healthier. The increased risk of lip, mouth and tongue cancer is equal to cigarette risk, even if you do not inhale.

◆ *Don't do anything to excess.*

Old wisdom, but true today. Excessive eating, drinking, smoking and even exercise can be harmful and expensive.

◆ *Make your home injury proof.*

Inspect your home for safety. Check electrical cords, the condition of carpeting, the placement of furniture and so on. Additions such as nonslip strips on bathtubs are inexpensive ways to ensure your safety and prevent the need for costly medical care.

◆ *Maintain a desirable weight.*

This does not necessarily mean that you should weigh what those famous charts say you should weigh, but you will be healthier if you weigh what feels good for you. And you'll save money on health care as well. Overweight people not only are more prone to conditions such as diabetes and heart disease, but they are also more likely to need hip, knee and other joint replacements in later years.

◆ *Wear seat belts.*

Some cars employ a passive restraint system that automatically fastens your seat belt; however, you may still need to manually fasten the lap belt. Whatever the case, you're always safer when you properly use the safety equipment that is included with your car. Forty-five thousand deaths a year, untold pain and suffering and loss of income should be enough to convince anyone to use seat belts.

◆ *Buy vehicles with air bags.*

Despite what you may have read about air bags, children and small adults, the overall record of air bags is excellent compared with seat belts alone. Thousands of lives that would otherwise have been lost have been saved (most without injury) by air bag deployment. As for children, they should always be restrained in the backseat, never the front. And be sure to always use your seat belt in conjunction with an air bag.

◆ *Always properly restrain children in cars.*

Remember: *You* are responsible for the safety of your children. It's a good idea to take along a car seat on airplanes and other forms of transportation. Injury prevention saves money and incalculable suffering. When using these re-straints, follow the printed instructions that come with the product. Not doing so will reduce the safety effectiveness of the product and could cause serious injury to your child.

◆ *Drive slower.*

Drivers who speed have more accidents than those who stay within the speed limits. Plus, don't be lured into thinking that the recent increase in speed limits in certain states is a license to jam down on the accelerator. Even those increased limits may be too fast for conditions. Be a little late, but arrive in one piece.

◆ *Avoid processed foods.*

Processed foods usually contain more fat, more salt and less fiber than unprocessed foods. They also contain preservatives and other chemicals. The healthier you are, the more money you will save on costly medical care—so pass the bran.

◆ *Have microwave emissions checked.*

Call the authorized repair service recommended in the literature accompanying your microwave. (Indeed, your manual should include a maintenance schedule.) A repair service should be able to do a quick, low-cost emission check. Microwave emissions are potentially harmful, so a few dollars for a check can save you medical costs in the future.

◆ *Purchase basic medical tools for self-diagnosis.*

You can save yourself time and expense by having basic medical tools such as a blood pressure cuff (sphygmoma-nometer), an otoscope (for looking in the ears) and a stetho-scope. Used in combination with a good medical guide, these tools can help you avoid many unnecessary visits to the doctor.

◆ *Join the People's Medical Society.*

The People's Medical Society *Newsletter* and our many other publications offer you an easy-to-read supply of medical information that you can use to make informed decisions about your health care.

◆ *Plan a fire escape route and hold home fire drills.*

Simple fire safety measures such as smoke alarms—an ample number placed strategically in your home—and fire drills can prevent serious injury or worse in the event of a home fire.

◆ *Exercise regularly.*

Regular exercise protects against heart disease, osteo-porosis and a variety of other common illnesses. It will also help you maintain a desirable weight and reduce stress. Joining a health club is cheaper than health care for a chronic illness such as heart disease.

◆ *Make friends and purchase a pet.*

Studies have shown that people who are socially active are healthier than those who are loners. Check your local newspaper for singles activities at churches, social organizations, Parents Without Partners, exercise clubs and so on. Place an ad in the personals section of newspapers and magazines or be daring and answer one!

Pets make great companions, and there are many dogs and cats at your local animal shelter just waiting for adoption. You'll have a lifelong friend and the satisfaction that comes with helping a less fortunate creature. How you feel mentally has long been known to be connected to how you feel physically, and being socially active and having a pet are two ways to improve your health. And remember that the cost for dog and cat food is considerably less than the cost of multiple doctor visits and prescription medications.

◆ *Wear a lead apron for dental x-rays.*

You should always shield the parts of your body not being x-rayed. Excessive radiation is a definite health hazard—and why invite trouble (and additional costs) when there's a simple remedy?

◆ *Keep current with immunizations.*

Adults need to be reimmunized periodically for tetanus and, in some areas of the country, other diseases as well. These immunizations often are given free or at a very low cost through community groups. Elderly adults and people with chronic conditions should consider immunization against influenza and pneumonia.

◆ *Avoid too much exposure to the sun.*

Dermatologists have definitely identified a link between exposure to the sun and skin cancer; however, you don't have to live in a cave. Use commonsense approaches to the sun: Always use a sunscreen with a sun protection factor (SPF) of 15 or more; keep your exposure to a minimum; don't get all your sun at once; and wear protective clothing such as a hat or long-sleeved shirt when in the sun.

For more information on how to enjoy the sun and avoid the hazards, contact

> Skin Cancer Foundation
> 245 Fifth Ave., Suite 1403
> New York, NY 10016
> 212-725-5176

◆ *Wash your hands.*

Frequent hand washing will lower your chances of catching colds, flu and other contagious diseases.

◆ *Take a vacation.*

Everyone needs and benefits from periodic breaks in the daily routine. Listen to yourself—don't get too burned out before you give yourself a break. Hotels are cheaper than hospitals.

◆ *Get enough sleep.*

Many conditions are related to or exacerbated by lack of sleep. Most people need seven to eight hours of sleep per day. Listen to yourself and make sure you get what you need.

◆ *Eat lots of fiber.*

Increasing the amount of fiber in your diet is the easiest way to lower your risk of colon cancer and heart attack. It will also help to lower cholesterol and prevent constipation.

Laxatives are much more expensive than an extra slice of whole-wheat bread.

◆ *Drink cranberry juice.*

Cranberry juice can be protective against bladder infections. But be careful to avoid the juices with a lot of added sugar and corn syrups. Cranberry juice is cheaper than antibiotics—and a lot more fun to ingest.

◆ *Brush your teeth and floss daily.*

Good oral hygiene is essential to good general health, so don't forget to brush and floss your teeth on a daily basis. Failure to develop and practice good oral health habits can be counterproductive to all your efforts at staying healthy. In addition, one unforeseen dental bill can wipe out any savings you've accumulated by practicing good general health.

Buy a plaque removal system for you and your family. Gum disease is one of the leading causes of tooth loss, and the cost to replace lost teeth can be quite high.

◆ *Contact a self-help support group.*

For many illnesses, a self-help support group can be as helpful as your doctor in speeding your recovery. Self-help support groups are in the business of empowerment, giving consumers the information and strategies they need to successfully deal with their conditions. In addition, in such groups, you meet people who share your condition and with whom you can share a common bond. For more information on self-help groups, contact

American Self-Help Clearinghouse
Northwest Covenant Medical Center
25 Pocono Rd.
Denville, NJ 07834
201-625-7101
201-625-9053 (TDD)

National Self-Help Clearinghouse
City University of New York
Graduate Center, Room 620
25 W. 43rd St.
New York, NY 10036
212-354-8525

◆ *Practice safe sex.*

Unfortunately and undeniably, sexually transmitted
diseases—gonorrhea, herpes, syphilis and human immuno-
deficiency virus (HIV, the virus that can cause AIDS), just to
name a few—are a nasty fact of life. Most at risk are those
people who have had many sexual partners. The risks,
however, are minimized if a condom is always and correctly
used during intercourse.

◆ *Know the number for your local*
poison control center.

Calling for help immediately if you suspect someone in
your family has ingested a poisonous substance can make the
difference between a minor digestive disturbance and a week
in the hospital's intensive care unit. Prompt action saves
lives and money.

◆ *Wear appropriate protective clothing and*
equipment when playing sports or engaging
in recreational activities.

Whether the activity is bicycling or football, protective
clothing can spare participants from easily preventable
injuries. Preventing injuries or lessening their severity
saves money.

GLOSSARY

Advance directive: A written document stating how a person wants medical decisions made for him if he is unable to make those decisions himself. The two most common advance directives are living wills and durable powers of attorney for health care.

Adverse reaction: A reaction that harms a person in some way.

Advocate: A person who represents another's interests.

Antihistamine: A medication used to treat allergy and cold symptoms such as itchy eyes and a runny nose.

Assignment: A process by which a doctor or hospital agrees to file an insurance claim in exchange for direct payment from the insurer. Under the Medicare system, the physician or hospital must also agree to accept that direct payment, plus any required patient copayments, as payment in full.

Audiologist: A health-care practitioner (non-M.D., non-D.O.) who specializes in treating hearing problems.

Balance billing: The practice of billing the patient for the difference between the doctor's usual charge and the amount paid by the insurance company.

Board certification (board certified): The status conferred upon a physician who has passed an examination given by a medical specialty board recognized by the American Board of Medical Specialists. Board certification is offered in 29 recognized specialties, such as pediatrics, obstetrics and gynecology and internal medicine.

Cesarean section (c-section): A method of delivering a baby by abdominal surgery.

Chiropractor: A health-care practitioner (D.C.; non-M.D., non-D.O.) who focuses on improving nerve function through manipulation and adjustment of body parts, particularly the spine.

Consultation: A discussion between physicians about a medical case or its treatment, for which the patient is billed.

Contraindication: Something that makes the use of a particular medication or treatment inadvisable.

Coordination of benefits: A review of benefit coverage done when two or more insurance plans cover the same procedure. The companies compare notes to determine who owes what. They split the bill, or at least the portion that is their responsibility, and the consumer must still pick up any copayment or deductible.

Copayment: A payment required of the patient in addition to the payment made by the insurance company. A copayment may be in the form of a deductible or a percentage payment (for instance, the insurance company pays 80 percent and the patient pays 20 percent).

Custodial care: The provision of room, board and personal services, generally on a long-term basis, without additional medical services.

Decongestant: A medication that acts to clear congestion. It helps such symptoms as stuffy nose or chest congestion.

Deductible: The amount a patient is required to pay before her insurance company begins to make payments.

Defensive medicine: The practicing of medicine with the goal of avoiding medical malpractice lawsuits, generally involving the ordering of many and perhaps unnecessary tests and procedures.

Diagnosis: The identification of a patient's illness through consideration of the signs and symptoms.

Durable power of attorney for health care: A form of medical advance directive that empowers a person to make health-care decisions for another should that person become unable to do so herself.

Family practitioner: A medical practitioner (M.D., D.O.) who specializes in treating the whole family, from uncomplicated births to care of the elderly.

Fee-for-service insurance plan: An insurance plan that reimburses the medical practitioner for services provided, in an amount that may or may not equal the charge of the procedure but which the practitioner agrees to accept as payment in full. The payment is generally sent directly to the practitioner.

Fellowship: A grant given to a medical practitioner that permits him to study a certain area of medicine, usually in conjunction with some specialty such as oncology or surgery. It may be used to develop direct patient-care modalities or for pure medical or biological research.

For-profit: A business that operates to make more money than it requires to continue operating.

General practitioner: A physician (M.D., D.O.) who can provide routine care for a wide range of medical problems.

Generic drug: A drug that is a copy of a brand-name drug. Its active ingredients must duplicate those of the brand-name drug.

Health maintenance organization (HMO): A form of managed care in which each consumer member pays a monthly premium in return for all necessary medical care. Members are covered only if they use doctors and medical facilities affiliated with the HMO and are subject to other restrictions as determined by their agreement. Costs incurred outside the network are usually not covered.

Homeopathic remedy: A medication used in homeopathy, which is a system of nontraditional medicine that is based upon the law of similars and the law of infinitesimals. The law of similars states that substances that provoke certain reactions in healthy people can be used to mitigate similar responses in people who are symptomatic. The law of infinitesimals states that the more vigorously a substance is diluted, the more potent it becomes.

Hospice: An organization that provides specialized care for dying patients either in their homes or at a special facility.

Indemnity insurance plan: An insurance plan that pays a set amount of reimbursement regardless of the fee charged by the practitioner. The insured is then responsible for payment of any excess charges. The payment is generally sent directly to the insured.

Interaction: The action of one drug upon the effectiveness or toxicity of another (or others).

Intermediate-care facility: A facility that provides less intensive care than a skilled nursing facility. Patients are generally more mobile, and rehabilitation therapies are stressed.

Internist: A physician (M.D., D.O.) who completes a three-year residency and passes a comprehensive examination but does not normally take training in pediatrics, orthopedics or child delivery. Instead, an internist has more advanced training in diagnosis and management of problems involving areas such as the gastrointestinal system, the heart, the kidney, the liver and the endocrine system.

Invasive treatment: A medical treatment that involves the invasion of the body with a drug or an instrument.

Itemized bill: A bill that lists each item and service and its corresponding charge.

Living will: A document that indicates a person's treatment wishes in the event that he is unable to verbally communicate those wishes. A living will is usually used as written authorization for the nonuse or removal of life-sustaining treatments.

Managed care: A form of health insurance that focuses on prevention, cost containment and the provision of high-quality health care to consumers through a defined network of practitioners and facilities.

Medicare and Medicaid HMOs: HMOs approved by the federal Health Care Financing Administration for Medicare and Medicaid beneficiaries' participation.

Midwife: See **Nurse-midwife**.

Nonparticipating physician: A physician that does not accept assignment. These physicians will bill for the cost of their services over the amount paid by insurance.

Nonprofit: An organization that functions by earning just enough money to continue operating.

Nosocomial infection: An infection acquired in the hospital.

Nurse practitioner: A nurse who has received specialized training that enables her to provide basic diagnostic medical care to patients.

Nurse-midwife: A medical practitioner who specializes in caring for women and delivering babies.

Open enrollment period: A period of time, defined by an insurer or health plan, during which anyone may apply for coverage and be accepted without evidence of insurability or waiting periods. The period may last from 30 to 90 days.

Open panel: A type of HMO in which private physicians are contracted by the HMO to provide services to its members. Under this model, the physician receives a monthly reimbursement for every HMO member who selects her practice, whether services are rendered or not. Most HMOs are open panel models.

Optometrist: A medical practitioner (O.D.) who specializes in examining eyes and who is able to prescribe corrective lenses but not perform surgery or invasive treatments.

Over-the-counter (OTC) drug: A drug that is available without a doctor's prescription.

Participating provider: A medical provider who has a contract with an insurer or health plan to provide services to covered persons and agrees to accept the reimbursement schedule of the plan as payment in full. The provider may be a physician, hospital, laboratory, outpatient facility or pharmacy.

Physician hospital organization (PHO): A managed-care plan owned by a hospital and the doctors affiliated with it.

Physician's assistant: A medical practitioner (P.A.) who is specially trained to provide a basic level of diagnostic medical care, usually under the supervision of a physician.

Physician's Desk Reference (PDR): A comprehensive reference book primarily listing prescription drugs and indications for use, contraindications and dosages.

Podiatrist: A medical practitioner (D.P.M.; non-M.D., non-D.O.) who specializes in caring for feet.

Point-of-service (POS) plan: A managed-care plan in which members pay monthly premiums for which they receive all the care they need from within the network of doctors and hospitals. If the member goes outside the network for care, the insurer still pays a significant portion of the bill. Out-of-pocket costs are capped.

Preferred-provider organization (PPO): A form of managed care, similar to an HMO, usually owned by the physicians. Costs outside the network are usually not covered.

Repackaging: The purchasing of products from a pharmaceutical distributor and then repacking of them into smaller units for sale under a different label.

Residency: A post-medical school training program, usually lasting from three to five years, in which a physician completes training in a speciality area, such as anesthesiology, emergency medicine or surgery. Completion of an approved residency program is a requirement for board certification.

Second opinion: An objective evaluation, diagnosis and treatment recommendation from a medical practitioner concerning a health problem that has previously been evaluated by another medical practitioner.

Side effect: An effect of a drug or treatment that is not directly a part of the healing process.

Skilled nursing facility: An institution that offers nursing services similar to those given in a hospital, to aid recuperation of those who are seriously ill.

Specialist: A doctor who concentrates on a specific body system, age group or disorder.

Staff model: A type of HMO in which the HMO actually employs its own physicians, paying each an annual salary and possibly a bonus.

Subspecialty: A specific area of medicine within a specialty. Usually, a specialist takes one or two more years of training to develop a subspecialty.